Into the Depths

A Chaplain's Reflections on Death, Dying and Pastoral Care

— ROSIE DEEDES —

Sacristy Press

Sacristy Press
PO Box 612, Durham, DH1 9HT

www.sacristy.co.uk

First published in 2019 by Sacristy Press, Durham

Sacristy Limited, registered in England & Wales, number 7565667

British Library Cataloguing-in-Publication Data
A catalogue record for the book is available from the British Library

ISBN 978-1-78959-032-6

This book is dedicated to my father Colin Deedes (1927–2013).

Contents

Acknowledgements

I am grateful to the people who have encouraged me to write, including my father Colin Deedes, and to others like Susi Bechhofer, Holocaust survivor, writer and personal friend, who inspired me. I am thankful to chaplaincy colleagues who read drafts of my first chapters and encouraged me to seek publication, and to my editor Natalie Watson who helped me shape my thoughts into this book.

I wrote some of the most emotionally challenging chapters whilst staying with the Sisters of Bethany in Southsea; I greatly appreciated the quiet and prayerful space that they provided for me to do so. I am indebted to all those people whose stories I have included and the many I have omitted; each has played a part in my formation as priest and pastor.

There have been many people who have sustained me in my ministry and to whom I am full of gratitude: counsellors, cell group members, colleagues, family and friends. My past and current spiritual directors and work supervisors, in particular, have helped me become more self-aware and enabled me to reflect on my work, emotionally, spiritually and theologically; I am indebted to each of them—Brother Bernard SSF, Duncan Ross, Muriel Green and Jane Edmunds.

My three children, Catherine, Hugh and Lucy, have enabled me to grow in the most life-affirming role of all and have provided me with the antidote to chaplaincy work—family life. Finally, to my generous husband, Jonathan Idle, who has educated our children, made homes wherever we have lived, and been a constant support to me. I have always had to hold firm boundaries between home and work life, and in reading drafts of this book he has found out more about my work than he has ever been able to find out before.

Introduction

This book has been a long time coming. As soon as I began working as assistant chaplain in Holloway women's prison in 1999, I knew that I wanted to write. The pastoral encounters were intense and rich with meaning, and I sensed they were worth sharing. The environment was unknown and unfamiliar to most people, so I felt that by writing I could educate people about prison and those who live and work there. I even had a title, *Pregnancy, Priesthood and Prison*. I was three months pregnant at the time. The book was going to be written during the quiet moments when my baby was fast asleep and I had the luxury of time to myself whilst on maternity leave. Needless to say, things didn't quite work out like that!

Two decades on, my firstborn is making her own way in the world, and my other two children are increasingly independent. I have moved from prison chaplaincy into hospice ministry, with a short exploration into university chaplaincy in between, and the book is about death rather than birth. The handful of pastoral encounters I could have talked about then have become hundreds, and the intervening years have hopefully given me greater insights and wisdom. I describe my journey through these various chaplaincy roles in Chapter 1.

Pastoral care has been fundamental to my ministry wherever I have worked. I would argue that it is the key component of all ministry, by ordained ministers or lay people, and by all those who offer care to others by listening compassionately. In Chapter 2 I unpack what exactly pastoral care is, and I discuss how pastoral care enables us to engage at depth with those we meet.

I have probably encountered more death and dying than most people would experience in several lifetimes. I use these experiences from my curacy, chaplaincy roles and family circumstances to reflect on what might be termed "good deaths" in Chapter 3; deaths which are particularly disturbing, including suicide, in Chapter 4; and deaths which might be described as "good enough" in Chapter 5. In Chapter 6 I discuss how I have accompanied those who have been bereaved. In Chapter 7 I consider the place and importance of rituals with people who are dying, or with the bereaved, focusing particularly on planning and conducting funerals.

In Chapter 8 I consider what I have needed to sustain myself to do this kind of ministry. I offer the wisdom gained from personal experience to those who are engaging at depth with others. Self-care and self-compassion are as important as care for others, and self-awareness helps to develop resilience and prevents getting burned-out or cynical.

In Chapter 9 I reflect on the taboo places where I have worked, prisons and a hospice, and the taboo subjects that these places prompt us to think about. I consider why it is important to break these taboos, and why it is also important to have a more informed, realistic and measured understanding of both kinds of environment.

This particular book could not have been written before I had gone through personal loss and grief. In 2013, in my last conversation with my father before he died, he encouraged me to write, but it has taken my move into the hospice to work to finally motivate myself to do so. The lessons I have taken from working with those who are dying, and which I explore in the final chapter, are that life is unpredictable, and death can come sooner than you anticipate. It is harder to die peacefully if you have regrets about things you have not done. So in 2018 I finally stopped procrastinating, and set myself the target of writing for publication, and this book is the result.

I write as a Christian and as a priest, and so the book is interwoven with passages from the Bible and the Christian tradition. I focus particularly on the stories of Jesus, and especially the last few days of his life, known as the Passion. It is my theological reflection on Jesus' own suffering which has helped me to face the suffering of others and to accompany them in it. It is my belief that in accompanying others into the depths, I have been spiritually and emotionally sustained by a loving God who has never left me. I could not have done this work without this faith.

Everything I have learned has come from those with whom I have travelled, in their imprisonments, their dying or grief. There are many whom I have not included, but each has played their part in my education. I am indebted to each of them. All names and some biographical details of the people I have described have been changed to maintain anonymity and confidentiality. Those whom I have been able to ask permission to tell their stories have been enthusiastic and generous in encouraging me to do so. They have said that if another person can learn something from the mistakes they made in life and so make different choices, then their life has had some purpose. Or if their experiences of facing death can help someone else face theirs with greater peace, then their dying has some meaning.

Giving someone the opportunity to express themselves and to be heard in a pastoral encounter can often help them to see their experiences in a new way, and gain a different perspective. This book seeks to do the same, to offer to the reader a fresh perspective on pastoral care, on prisons and on death itself. I hope it will promote thought and discussion about subjects which most of us prefer to avoid, but which, when we look at them in a new way, become less frightening and taboo.

Much of this book has been written as I have sat in the bay window of my bedroom, looking out over wonderful sea views. It is by looking outward, and beyond, towards the horizon, that I have been helped to maintain my own sense of perspective. On a rather cloudy and windy day recently my eleven-year-old daughter and I were watching the heavy dark clouds chasing across the sky and seeing shafts of sunlight breaking through them, streaming spots of bright light onto the sea below. With our binoculars we followed the struggles of a small yacht battling the rough grey seas and heading towards a patch of sunlight. I commented that the people on the boat, when it reached the light, would not know that it was in it, and that it is only from our position that we could see it. It is all about perspective. My daughter remarked that I should include that in this book; a commentary on life and death perhaps, so I have.

CHAPTER 1

Into the Depths

In my work in prisons, and a hospice, I have frequently seen people who have been in the depths of despair, and as chaplain I have offered them companionship and pastoral care. In this opening chapter I describe chaplaincy operating in different secular contexts—prisons and hospice—and how chaplains stand on the edge of the Church institution. I reflect on the personal challenges of working with many victims of sexual violence (women in prison) and then with perpetrators (male sex offenders) and of working with death daily. I use pastoral experiences to illustrate these challenges. I consider some of the psychological pitfalls and projections onto chaplains, and the importance of self-awareness as protection against these dangers.

Chaplain on the edge

I visited Kelly every day when I was on duty in the prison. She would never respond, and her face was turned towards the wall. She was sometimes on the floor, curled up in a foetal position, dressed in the prison issue outfit that was supposed to be indestructible. If she had worn anything else, she would have torn it up to make a ligature and tried to hang herself. There was a member of staff outside her door constantly to make sure she didn't make any further suicide attempt. Frequently she had pulled out her catheter and would be lying in a pool of her own urine. She couldn't move about her own cell, except by shuffling along; a previous suicide attempt had left her paralysed in the lower part of her body, and she had no use of her legs. I greeted her through the hatch of her door, saying simply, "Hello Kelly, I know you don't want to talk at the moment, but I am here if and when you do." Then I would stay for a few minutes, say farewell and tell her I would see her the next day. This continued for weeks.

A painting of the Gospel story in John 4, by Sieger Köder, depicts a woman standing at a well, looking into the depths below. As a chaplain in prisons for women and men, as a university chaplain, and currently as a hospice chaplain, I have frequently stood on the edge of the well, looking into the depths of human suffering, despair and misery. Sometimes, as with Kelly, the depths have been visible right there in front of me; at other times it is when someone has disclosed in conversation the pain of grief, abuse, an offence, a broken relationship. Sometimes they have not really known what they were going to tell me when they first came into my office, or I met them in a corridor, but as the conversation has continued and the trust has developed, they have felt more able to unburden their souls, knowing now that I would not judge them, but would only listen. It is one of the most humbling and moving experiences to listen, not only to the words that are expressed but to the physical and emotional pain that someone is carrying.

Many times, I have been the first person they have told about their experience, and the risk of doing so is great. Will I blame them? Will I condemn them? Will I tell them off? Will I believe them? Perhaps they have tried to tell others before but have not really been heard. Perhaps they have tried to tell others before and not been believed. Perhaps others have said, you should be over it by now; it can't have been as bad as all that; pull yourself together. Sadly, these are the kind of things that people will have experienced by the time they come to tell their story to a chaplain. Many times, I have felt in myself great sorrow; my eyes have misted over. Sometimes I have felt anger welling up inside at the injustice I am hearing about. In these moments I have an internal dialogue: "This is not my pain, this is not my story." Sometimes I have had to dig my nails into the palms of my hands, to remind me that there is a difference between my own physical pain and theirs. "I must not let my own emotional reaction to what I am hearing take over. I am here just to bear witness. God—you have got to help me out here. This is such a hard place to be right now." The woman in Köder's painting sees her own reflection in the water, and alongside it, the face of Jesus. I have looked deep into the well of human misery and have also seen Jesus' face, and felt his presence with me. I could only bear to do so, knowing that Jesus was somehow in the suffering, and with me witnessing it.

As a chaplain I have always been on the edge, not just of sorrow and grief, but also of the Church. I think as chaplains this is where we are meant to be. Comfortable on the edge of organized religion, and at home with those on the edge of society; perhaps this is a good definition of a chaplain? As a child of the vicarage I cannot claim to have experienced abject poverty, homelessness or abuse. I have lived in comfortable homes, in pleasant places, and attended schools which gave me a good education. I have only known warmth, affection and love from those around me, but I have been drawn throughout my life to those who have not had the advantages that I have had, or who by virtue of circumstance find themselves in a difficult situation. Perhaps this is the guilt of the affluent and secure, and could be considered patronizing or paternalistic, but I hope it is something else.

As a Christian, I feel very drawn to the person of Jesus, and to his ministry. In him I find someone who felt most at ease with those who were either outcast from society, or on its edge—lepers, blind people, "sinners", rather than those who were self-righteously religious and "good". My upbringing and education gave me access to the Christian story, and the gospel message, and it is my attempt to live in response to this that has taken me into chaplaincy.

Chaplaincy and the Church

I have an ambivalence about the Church. In many ways it has nurtured me, shaped my theology and faith, educated me and enabled me to live a role where I can be fully myself. It has for a short period of my adult life paid my wages and given me a home. There have been times when I have experienced a church congregation as a wonderful community of diverse people giving love and acceptance to one another and representing all the aspirations of the kingdom of God. But there have been other times when I have despaired of the Church, and my own branch of it—the Church of England. I have seen it as an exclusive and excluding place, which exists for the benefit of perpetuating itself, rather than preaching the gospel message. I have heard mission talked of when really it is fund-raising, and I have seen decisions made in the name of Jesus, which I am convinced would make him weep!

In chaplaincy I often encounter people who are "un-churched" or "once-churched". I have probably heard from more people who have lost faith because they have been hurt by the church than people who have found peace within it. However, I am also aware that a church is a gathered community of people who know their need of God, that they are as sinful, self-centred and flawed as anybody else, and that they, like everyone else, are works in progress. No one who comes to church should expect perfection! What they should expect is welcome, acceptance, honesty, forgiveness and love. Sadly, people sometimes confuse the Church with God, and so by dismissing the Church, they dismiss God as well. I try to reassure people that the two are not synonymous and that God is far greater than organized religion, and that Jesus did not come to establish an institution.

This is one of the fundamental differences between chaplaincy and parish ministry. As parish priest or minister, you will primarily deal with people with a common set of beliefs who come together with a similar purpose. You are perceived as a leader of a group of people, having a certain standing within the local community, with particular responsibilities and tasks to perform, and people approach you in this role. As a chaplain I mostly meet people at a point of need, who may or may not have any contact with a church; they could have a faith or belief which is completely different to my own; they could be highly suspicious of me or what I appear to represent to them; they could tell me politely or not that I am not welcome.

As a chaplain one is invited into an institution such as a hospice or prison. Frequently we are paid employees like everyone else. We do the same training, work to the same principles and are managed within the structures of the organization, often by people who have no religious or faith background themselves. The job we are employed to do, for example as managing chaplain in a prison, would be open to any Christian denomination or any faith leader who met the criteria and was successful at interview. The job could have been offered to a Pagan, a Muslim or a Humanist. This is so completely different to ministry in a parish or church, where, in the Church of England, each post will only be open to a person of that denomination, where people of the local church will have a say in the appointment, along with the bishop and the senior clergy of the diocese. Once in post a parish priest has complete autonomy, is left to get on with the job as they see fit, and is subjected to little oversight or management.

To become a chaplain having been used to working in a parish setting is a challenge for many; it requires a relinquishing of authority and power and accepting with humility the constraints that others in the organization must work with. It is a fine balance for ordained ministers working in chaplaincy to keep their sense of vocation and calling within a model of secular employment. Should I count my hours like others employed, or should I work over and above these because of my vocation? I have always wrestled with a sense of guilt that I have had two days off a week as a chaplain, on a par with those who work alongside me, whereas fellow priests in parish settings generally have only one.

In church-based ministry a priest or minister in charge of a church is like a big fish in a small pond; they will be involved in all decision-making. In chaplaincy this is very different. In a university a chaplain is a tiny minnow. In a church the congregation has expectations of their minister and some understanding of what clergy do; in chaplaincy immediate colleagues and managers may have little idea about what we do, why we do it, or how it can contribute to the organization or to the lives of the community. Managers may even be hostile to chaplaincy and seek to impose or over-manage what we do, disregarding the professional expertise with which we come to ministry. This can be a painful and lonely position to be in, so good support, supervision and connecting with other chaplains can be vitally important and sustaining.

Chaplains may have to justify their position in a secular institution. They may be required to give evidence and proof of the monetary value of what they bring. Their hours could be cut when the organization faces financial constraints, and there may be few who will speak up for us. Will you increase the number of chaplains or nurses in a hospital setting? Chaplains have little power within the organization but they can be afforded a degree of moral authority because of their role as faith leaders.

Prison governors have frequently referred to chaplaincy as the conscience of the organization, and I have been thanked by senior managers, when I was part of the senior management team, for presenting another side, often a more humane one, to a contentious discussion.

In parish ministry the liturgical role of the priest or minister will be central, and Sunday worship the one occasion where the community expects to see the minister; in chaplaincy, it is the pastoral role that is always of primary importance. Liturgy and worship are a much smaller part of what we do but always arise out of pastoral necessity. In some cases, as in my experience as a university chaplain, there was no expectation of a liturgical role for the chaplain, and I worked a normal working week, Monday to Friday.

In many ways the chaplaincy model is more like the deacon's position, that of servant and service. Chaplains are present to serve the community, not of believers, but the wider community associated with the location; be it hospice, prison or university. People I meet often ask me if I have a church in addition to the chaplaincy role I am doing, as if this is where a person in a collar should be, not in a secular environment where they are out of place. I don't worry about this any more. I probably wouldn't want to be constrained by the expectations of the institutional Church. I fear I would be hopelessly inadequate to the task. However, I do feel passionately that the model of chaplaincy where we are on the outside of the church organization; where we represent the love of God through our compassion and engagement with people at a point of need; where we relinquish the power of position by being in a secular environment; is one that has much to teach the rest of the established Church.

Chaplaincy in women's prisons

Towards the end of my compulsory three-year curacy in a parish, I began to wonder where I ought to go next. Many of the contemporaries with whom I had trained were moving into parishes, and yet I never felt this was where my gifts could best be used. The one and only clergy residential I attended as a curate was to shape the next sixteen years in ministry. There I met the chaplain to HMP Holloway. I was interested in his work and asked if I might visit him there, as I had never been to a prison before. He agreed, and when I went there to meet him on that first occasion, I immediately felt at home. It seemed to be the kind of environment where I could be fully myself; a "no holds barred" sort of place, similar in many respects to working with people who are homeless, as I had done in my curacy; with them, too, there is no standing on ceremony and people will tell you exactly how it is.

Working with women in prison is emotionally demanding, intensely challenging, very real, and I loved it. I had no idea until I met people in other parts of the prison service that so many prison staff would shy away from working in a prison with women. Many people would say to me, "I don't know how you could do it, you wouldn't get me working with women." Women make up about five per cent of the overall prison population, so by coming to work here I was choosing a minority group within an already-marginalized organization. Holloway had a certain notoriety about it. It has held high-profile women prisoners, and at times in its history has had a terrible reputation for the conditions and the behaviour of the prisoners, and sometimes staff.

I have considered why people were so fearful of, or resistant to, working with women in prison. In part I believe it is because women who have committed offences are seen to have broken and violated the rules of womanhood and mothering; somehow, they are presented as more dangerous by having done so. I think also people see women in prison as loud, confrontational and questioning of the rules, whereas men in prison are more compliant. Certainly, most women are more overtly emotional and often experience the pain of being in prison differently to men. Their primary concern on coming to prison is for their children. The social cost of imprisoning women is often greater as women are frequently the carers of children, so when they come to prison the family disintegrates, whereas when a father comes to prison, there is often a mother keeping a family intact.

Most people who go into prison for the first time will have fears, preconceptions and anxieties about being in this environment. Their families will also share these concerns. While I had felt entirely comfortable after my first visit to prison, some of my family were very concerned about my working there. My parents would have preferred to see me in almost any other kind of chaplaincy than prison. They thought that it would not be safe, and that I would see and hear some terrible things; they may have doubted my ability to cope. Looking back from the vantage point of being a parent myself, I have a better understanding of their concerns for me. Their anxieties were even greater when I told them that I would be starting the job when I was three months pregnant.

I was choosing to enter a prison; I would be carrying keys; I knew that I would be leaving there every evening, that I would have a specific role and responsibilities, that I would be supported by a team of colleagues, and that I could hand in my notice if it didn't work out. Prisoners coming to a prison have no such reassurances, and nor do their families. Many prisoners coming to Holloway would also have been pregnant and would have also worried about the safety of their unborn children.

After less than a week in the prison, I had already recognized that the experiences I encountered were profoundly challenging—pastorally, and emotionally. I felt exhausted and close to tears at the end of the day. Perhaps the newness of the environment and the harshness of the location exacerbated what anyone would feel in a new role. I was struck particularly by the needs of the women for instant gratification. The demands of women, particularly those who are detoxing from drugs or alcohol, were immense. If they wanted a rosary, or a radio, they wanted it now. I also felt the enormous physical and psychological burden of carrying keys. Wearing a substantial belt with a bunch of keys on a chain in a pouch is what I imagine it must be like to wear a chastity belt! Even normal activities such as using the toilet are more complicated by the baggage you carry around your waist. This was particularly challenging when I was pregnant—as my pregnancies progressed, it was difficult to know whether to put the belt above or below the bump!

The physical environment of Holloway was also challenging. There were innumerable stairs, and long corridors to negotiate, and I found often that I might go to a particular wing to see someone who had requested a visit, only to find that they had moved or were at some activity, and I would have to return later. Prisons are not places of beauty. Some may have nice gardens which are a pleasant relief to those who reside there as well as the staff. But generally, they are functional, grey and inhospitable buildings. Holloway felt to me particularly so. The place had a general air of being ill-cared-for and a poor environment to work in. And for those who had to live there, it must have felt even more so. For women who were coming into prison for the first time, who were already in a state of shock, adapting to these circumstances was incredibly difficult. There is much emphasis on the need to support prisoners on their first night in custody, to prevent them from being overwhelmed completely.

What was particularly striking was the noise. There is no quiet anywhere in a busy local prison. The doors bang loudly; the keys rattle in the locks; the staff raise their voices to be heard amongst the chatter. The women shout. Even when I was in my office at lunchtime, and all the women were locked in their rooms—on "patrol state"—the women would be shouting to one another from one part of the prison to the next. Whole conversations, expressing love or hate, could be conducted in this manner, without anyone seeming to mind the fact that hundreds of others could hear. Some of these conversations could be quite touching, when one woman expressed care or concern for another. Sometimes they seemed pretty abusive, threatening and aggressive; frequently the language was very coarse. But sometimes it could be humorous too. Once I heard this shouted out the window by a convicted arsonist: "How do you turn a jacket into a blazer? Set light to it at the edges!"

Most people will form an impression of women in prison, or any prisoner, based on the presentation in the media as well as prejudice and ignorance. What I discovered, in eleven years of working in women's prisons, was the depth of vulnerability, the complicated life-stories, and the resilience of many of the women who ended up there. Contrary to public misconceptions, most women in prison were not violent, but were mostly in prison for acquisitive crimes, to do with funding or maintaining an addiction. Many of the women reported horrendous experiences of abuse, physical, sexual, emotional. Most were mothers, and several had such chaotic lifestyles that their children had been taken into care.

In any women's prison there was a substantial contingent of foreign national women, many of whom were convicted of drug importation. These women were mostly "mules" carrying drugs in their luggage, or on their person, either externally or internally. Some women had been duped by drug dealers to carry these substances, being promised financial rewards for doing so. They were told that if caught they would be sent back to their homeland. This might have been the case, but only after many years in custody. Many of these women were from impoverished backgrounds, seeking to pay school fees for their children or hospital fees for elderly parents. Some brought in drugs unknowingly, but since this could never be proved their sentences reflected the weight of drugs smuggled and rarely paid any heed to the story behind it. The vast majority of these women were in prison for the first time. Often, they had left children behind and were beside themselves at what would happen to them. The experiences of these women were heart-breaking.

As chaplains we visited all those who had come into the prison within the last twenty-four hours. Often, we saw women in shock, having come straight from court or a police cell. They had been through the reception experience when we saw them, which had required them to be strip- searched and given the prison issue items to see them through the first hours in custody. One foreign national woman had left behind an infant she was still breast-feeding. She was in agony physically from her engorged breasts, as well as emotionally from the reality of the separation which lay before her. As a mother of a young baby myself, whom I was also breast-feeding, I felt a physical reaction to her pain and grief.

Some foreign-national women, on discovering that they would be in prison for a long time, would keep the reality of their situation from their families; they might tell children or parents that they were away working or studying. Sometimes the strain of keeping up this façade was immense, but the shame of admitting the truth outweighed the pain. I cannot imagine what psychological harm was done to young children both by this experience of separation and by keeping the truth from them.

I found that women in prison were incredibly forthcoming about themselves, their lives and their emotions. In Holloway each day we had an intake of up to thirty new prisoners, all of whom needed to be seen by a chaplain. There was not enough time to see everyone whilst they were out of their cells, so we had to talk to some of them through a hatch when they were locked in their cell. Within a few minutes of meeting a chaplain, a woman was likely to have poured out her story and shared her feelings. They were often incredibly grateful for the opportunity to do so, to someone like myself who showed compassion and was able to listen with kindness. I had nothing else to offer each woman. I could do nothing to change her situation or to ease her sorrow, but frequently the woman would begin to regain her humanity and a sense of her own worth because she felt listened to and reassured.

As a female chaplain working with women there was a bond of connectedness between myself and the prisoners. I had all three of my children while I was working in women's prisons, and I found the women, most of whom were mothers themselves, were delighted to share with me their advice and guidance about my pregnancies and child-rearing. It was a point of real shared experience, and for many of the women it was an opportunity to show me kindness and care. It gave them a sense of worth that they had something to offer which I was able to receive and welcome. The women's interest in my children continued, and despite the sadness of separation from their own families, they were generously able to show an interest in mine. I found this very humbling.

In any prison there is a high proportion of prisoners with mental illness. The environment and circumstances can lead many to become depressed and suicidal, but often prisoners come to prison with a long history of psychological disturbance. Women prisoners, who make up 5 per cent of the prison population, account for 50 per cent of reported incidents of self-harm. Self-harm comes in many forms—cutting, burning, food refusal and suicide attempts. In Holloway in particular there were countless alarm bells for incidents, many of which involved women making serious attempts to inflict pain on themselves. Staff in prison had to witness and deal with some horrendously distressing situations, often in quick succession. It is a challenging place to work and it is not surprising that it has an impact on the attitudes and behaviours of those who do so.

Working with staff in prison

I have always spent much of my time in prison working with and listening to staff. I met some who clearly loathed the job and talked of the prisoners as "cons" (convicts, though many in Holloway were on remand, so were technically innocent until proven guilty). Some staff thought the regime too soft; others felt that prisoners didn't know how good they had it, and that the prisoners should be grateful to the staff for all that they do. Others had come into the service to change the world, to make a difference to the lives of the women or men inside by treating them with respect and humanity.

When I first arrived in Holloway, I felt some staff were checking me out by their comments, to see whether I was soft and fluffy, and likely to be taken for a ride by the more unscrupulous prisoners. In my first week I had a very challenging conversation with a somewhat hardened female officer. It seemed she was really testing me out to see my reactions. She said that not everyone who had been abused ended up in prison, and that these "cons" were all losers. She also remarked that the demand for rosaries and Bibles from chaplains, and the numbers of people coming to the chapel, was nothing to do with their faith.

If you didn't come to chapel on a Sunday at Holloway, you would probably be locked up, because there were insufficient officers to staff the services and keep the wings open. In 1999, when I began as chaplain, there was no in-cell electricity, so if you were locked in your cell, there was no TV, and unless you had tiny battery-operated radios lent by the chaplains, you were without distraction. No wonder the women opted for chapel! I am sure that many of the women treated faith like a superstition, and I told the officer this. But as chaplains and people of faith, we start where people are, and we are not in the business of measuring outcomes. I have always looked at my role in chaplaincy as being like a sower, sowing seeds, and only God sees the growth. I wonder what seeds were sown through that particular conversation with a staff member.

What was my role with staff? To listen, and not to judge, to understand without condemning. I felt right from the start of my time in prison that is was important to challenge the division and separation of "us and them", and to demonstrate in action and word my belief that we all share a common humanity, and there but for the grace of God could be any of us, on the other side of the prison bars. I felt the need to counteract cynicism and to provide alternative explanations for the behaviours of prisoners. The necessity to challenge these attitudes in staff remained with me throughout my time in prison, and although I built constructive and affirming relationships with many members of staff, there were always some who I felt had either been in the job too long, or who should never have started in it. Negativity in that kind of environment is understandable when the pressures on staff are so great, when resources are scarce, and when the public is constantly critical or oblivious of what you do. I felt that as chaplain I tried to bring a sense of value to the role of the staff, to affirm them in the complexity of what they had to manage every day, but at the same time to encourage them to hold on to the view of each prisoner's humanity.

As chaplain within a prison there are clear expectations of what you will do. These are statutory duties: visiting all the prisoners who had just arrived, seeing all the prisoners in the hospital wing, and visiting the segregation unit (wing where prisoners are held for punishment or for their own protection). These are daily tasks and are measurable actions that are recorded in a chaplain's journal. In addition, there are expectations that a chaplain will break bad news of a relative's death to a prisoner, and that they will be available to prisoners for pastoral support when requested. While many people working in prisons show care to prisoners, they are always mindful of the boundaries which need to be maintained. Prisoners are sometimes reluctant to trust prison staff and may feel more comfortable speaking to a chaplain whom they see in a different light.

Chaplaincy with male sex offenders

I loved working with women in prison, perhaps because there was a natural bond of womanhood which made it possible for me to be myself. I was able to share at a very personal level their life stories, most of which contained tragedy and loss. It is a well-recorded fact that many of the women in prison have been victims themselves of abuse, and for some coming to prison was respite from the violence. Perhaps there is something in my make-up which looks for new challenges and does not want to get complacent or stale; and after eleven years of working with women and eight in the same prison, Downview, I began to consider what I should do next. I knew of a vacancy at a HMP Albany on the Isle of Wight, a beautiful location to live, but it would mean working in a prison for male sex offenders. You cannot hear story after story of domestic or child abuse from women in prison without forming strong views about perpetrators. This was going to be my new community to work amongst; given all that I had heard and thought about for so long, this was going to be a challenge indeed.

I had to work hard on myself, and my approach to life, to make this shift. Was I really as non-judgemental as I liked to think I was? Was I betraying the women I had supported and helped to empower with self-belief by working with the kinds of men who had caused them so much harm? Would I be safe myself in this environment? It was indeed a testing time of inner wrestling. Those questions stayed with me throughout the five years I was there, but I learned from those with whom I worked so much again about life and myself.

On my first day in the new prison I was shown round by an officer from the security department. I was wearing a skirt. It was long, straight and smart, but it had a split in the front seam. The officer advised me not to wear a skirt like that. I felt incredibly naïve and foolish, as well as uncomfortable. I wondered what kind of environment I had come to. I don't think I ever wore a skirt to work again. On another occasion I was wearing boots with a slight heel, and a prisoner made some comment—they were consigned to the cupboard for ever! This sort of thing I had never had to think about in the women's prison, but a long-term male prison is another experience altogether. I missed the camaraderie of female colleagues in the women's estate; there were women officers, nurses and governors in the prison, but they were very few in number, and there was a much more macho culture amongst the staff in the male estate than I was used to.

Albany Prison had a long corridor from which the residential wings branched off. When meals were served, the prisoners would queue along this corridor to collect their food from the servery. I used to have to steel myself to walk along this route when all the prisoners were gathered; a conspicuous female figure wearing a clerical shirt attracted attention which I was never comfortable with. Many of the men in this kind of prison had a very poor image and understanding of women generally, and several were not used to women in positions of authority or leadership. My natural manner is gentle and quietly spoken, so some of the staff thought I would be a soft touch and would struggle to survive in that environment. Just as I had been challenged when I first arrived in Holloway, so I had to win the trust and confidence of the staff in Albany, and the other Isle of Wight prisons which became one establishment during my time there. My maxim for prison work has always been to "be wise as serpents and innocent as doves" (Matthew 10:16b). There is no doubt that when I started in Albany, I felt that I was being sent out like a sheep in the midst of wolves (Matthew 10:16).

I did not change my persona working with this new client group, but it was never as comfortable a working environment as it had been in the women's estate. I had to completely separate my home life and work life. I could not discuss at home anything that happened in the prison. It became like a double life, which, ultimately, I found unbearable. Being a priest and pastor means bringing yourself into the role; that is hard to do when you cannot tell those with whom you work even the vaguest details about your family life. This was a sharp contrast to my experience in women's prisons. My father died while I was chaplain in HMP Isle of Wight, and whereas in more normal circumstances of a parish, or even in a women's prison, the congregation would have prayed for him and for me, and would have known what was happening, I could not disclose anything about it in the context of this new prison. I think it was at this point that I began to feel that for my own wellbeing it was time to move on to something else.

I discovered that I was able to have compassion for the male prisoners, and to approach them without judgement. I have always believed that people in prison have already been judged by the courts and judicial system. It is not for me to judge them further but to support them as they face their situation and themselves. I learned that many of the men had also experienced abuse or deprivation of love and affection, and whereas I had found that more women internalized their abuse and self-harmed, men more often fought back and acted in the same way to others as they had experienced themselves. I saw the tragedy of human existence and abuse from every angle. What I have always tried to do with anyone I have encountered, whom I have found particularly challenging, is to try and see them as I believe God sees them—through the eyes of love and compassion. I also believe that no one was born evil, and that it is our circumstances and life experiences from a very early age which shape our choices and who we become. There were some I found difficult to like, whom I pictured as small children, before they had inflicted such harm on others.

There was one particular prisoner I can recall who brought this home to me. He was a strange individual, quite a loner, with mental health issues and addictions, whom I was advised to be wary of. I rarely read the full history of someone's offence, but I was always aware of enough to be safe when with them. This individual, Paul, had had a history of violence against women including rape. Somehow, we managed to build a rapport, and together we explored issues of spirituality and faith. He felt drawn to Buddhism but was also interested in the Gospels. I sensed he had burdens from his past that he needed to talk about. He had begun to recognize the distorted image he had of women, and to trace this back to his early life experiences. He had been repeatedly abused by his elder sister and her boyfriend and aged five had been engaged in sexual activity with them both. These acts had been filmed and shown to his wider family. His father then called him a monster, and the rest of his life he had been living up to this image. In the course of our conversations Paul alluded to other offences which he had committed and for which he had never been caught. He felt the burden of them for his victims, and eventually he disclosed these and was convicted and transferred to a high security prison as a result. This was probably the first noble, empathetic act and positive choice Paul had made throughout his unhappy, loveless and dysfunctional life. I hope it was the start of a journey to some healing, but I will never know.

Some of the most challenging prisoners to work with were those who denied their sexual offences. There was one woman whose case was still high-profile in the media, who insisted that she had done no wrong. It was hard to separate what was being said about her in the press from the image she conveyed in the prison. She also expressed a strong faith, and she would request to speak to members of the chaplaincy team and ask for prayers for her release. It is a fine balance to tread between honesty, collusion and compassion. In these circumstances I could only reiterate that God alone knows the truth of any of our situations, and pray to God who reveals the secrets of our own hearts, "Thy will be done."

At HMP Isle of Wight, which held mostly sex offenders, there were many more prisoners who denied the charges they were accused of. It is the policy of the prison service that the decision of the court is accepted, and if the prisoner feels wrongly accused, they must use the legal process to appeal. This gave me permission to work with the prisoner based on the reality of their situation and not to be drawn into the question of their innocence or guilt. Denial is complex; for some it is a protection from the horror and reality of what they are capable of; for some it is a way of presenting themselves in a more positive light to family, friends or themselves; for some it is a matter of interpretation of circumstances—was the sexual encounter with consent or not? For some it is a distorted sense of what is acceptable and right. I recall sitting with a prisoner who told me directly that he refused to accept the term "paedophile", which had been used of him by the courts because he had only had sex with his under-age step-daughter in his own home!

It is all-consuming working in prisons, and those who work there can become as institutionalized as those who live there. Working with sex offenders, even when one tries to be non-judgemental and open-minded, is difficult, as some prisoners can be manipulative and controlling. There are psychological and sub-conscious dangers of working in this kind of environment for too long – it may be hard to switch off from prisoners' crimes; one may become over-suspicious of the behaviour of the general public; or imagine that everyone is a sexual predator; relationships between prison staff and their partners may be negatively affected. I have known prison staff report feeling angry with family members, and their relatives reporting that they treat their children like they do the prisoners. There are practical constraints too; in a prison every door is locked and every implement accounted for—there can be carry-over from work to home with this sort of anxiety. I did not want to get to the stage where these issues were affecting me adversely and impacting on my family.

Chaplaincy in a hospice

The working environment of a hospice is very different to a prison. Although some people will have the same reservations about coming to a hospice as prisoners may feel about coming to prison, the layout, atmosphere and physical environment is designed to be welcoming, homely, beautiful and relaxing. I cannot imagine a prison being designed along these lines.

The ethos of the hospice is to provide compassionate care to anyone who comes there, as patient, family member or visitor. All the staff and volunteers are committed to that. People often remark that the hospice has a particular atmosphere which they cannot quite describe, but which makes them feel at ease. There are no locked doors, minimal security, and free movement around the hospice. In the Mountbatten Hospice, where I now work, there is an art gallery as well as a café and chapel and beautiful gardens to walk around. The attractiveness of the environment mitigates perhaps the fear of dying. Many come to the hospice expecting it to be a place of gloom and despondency; they are surprised.

As a chaplain in a hospice there are no specific tasks or daily activities which must be undertaken. It is a much smaller working environment than a prison; with sixteen beds in the inpatient unit, it is more the size of a hospital wing in a prison. By wandering around the inpatient unit of the hospice I can meet with patients and their families casually and build up a rapport with them. Some chaplains may adopt the approach of seeing all the patients every day, like the prison model, but I have chosen to be guided by the nursing staff as to who they think would like a visit on any particular day. As staff have learned to trust me in the hospice they now feel confident to ask me to visit a particular patient whom they feel might be in some kind of spiritual or emotional distress or just in need of a conversation.

My personal preference for chaplaincy work is to be spontaneous and flexible. I have always valued the opportunity to "loiter with intent", to be around in places where I am visible and approachable to those who might wish to have a conversation. In prison this would mean hanging around at meal times, or when prisoners are returning from work to their wings; in the hospice, it means having lunch in the dining area of the day patients' unit, or sitting in the nurses' office having a cup of tea.

The dangers of chaplaincy

There are dangers of working in chaplaincy, but perhaps not the kind that people would automatically expect. When I worked in prisons, people often asked if I was ever frightened or if I had been attacked. I always felt physically safe in prison, and was never attacked myself, though I did witness violence on a few occasions. There are psychological dangers of chaplaincy that require self-awareness and humility to unpack.

There are the "ego-dangers" of working in extreme circumstances; those who do not work in these settings might project onto you the "hero" or the "angel". They may say things like, I don't know how you can work in those places; I could never do it. It must be so sad, or so demanding, or so frightening. Immediately there is the danger of the internal voice within me saying, "You are special, you are better than other people." The temptation of these projections is to let them feed your ego until you believe them. Bursting the ego bubble is vital to maintain integrity and sanity: failure to do so can lead to the mistaken belief that you are indispensable to the organization, or to the world.

In the hospice world the pitfalls are probably even greater than in the prison. I find as chaplain I am more in the public eye and exposed to a greater range of people. There is much more feedback from those I work with about what I do, and generally it is positive. Whether that is my taking a funeral or being with a family at a deeply significant moment of their lives, people will often express their gratitude for my involvement. Even when a member of staff says, "You are always smiling", or "You are such a good listener", I am aware and wary of my psychological reaction to them. How tempting to then see myself in these terms—to crave this kind of attention and feedback to ensure that I am doing a good job and living up to the expectations of others. How pressurizing though, to need to be "practically perfect in every way" like Mary Poppins!

I am more aware of these traps and follies in my fifties than I was in my thirties when I set out in ministry. What has kept me grounded have been the people in my life who have seen my flaws and follies and loved me just the same. My husband and my children have been the greatest antidote to the projections of other people. Children at any age see through pomposity, self-importance and falsity, and require you to be yourself. They help you to laugh at yourself should you need encouragement to do so. Wise people who mirror back to you your strengths and weaknesses, and who love you with both, are essential to gather around you to mitigate the disasters of over-exalted egos. I am less bothered now by how I am perceived by others, as I become more and more comfortable and honest with myself.

These psychological dangers are probably found in any kind of ministry, particularly where one is seen to carry some moral authority or weight by wearing a clerical shirt. I have seen people seek to put clergy onto pedestals (probably to knock them off at some point later!). I have observed this from the vantage point of a child of a clergyman. I have always tried to resist this myself, and perhaps that is why I chose to move into the more hidden world of prison chaplaincy. Prisoners perhaps throw different projections at you—that you are a soft touch; that you are going to talk about God all the time; that you will be easily offended by swearing; that you don't have sex! Generally, prisoners tell you it as it is and keep you firmly grounded in the mess, muddle and grittiness of human experience, where being honest, having integrity and being authentic are crucial components of meaningful relationships and ministry. I am indebted to them.

Chaplaincy and death

Chaplains in any context become a valuable resource to a secular organization when there is a death or serious incident; whether that is breaking bad news about a death of a contemporary to prisoners or to cohorts of students, or informing an individual prisoner of the death of a relative. It might be leading a memorial service for a member of staff who has died, or facilitating some act of remembrance after a catastrophic world event; in these circumstances managers and individuals will look to the chaplain to do something. We are considered to have expertise, skills and qualities that enable us to deal with the emotional and psychological distress associated with death and dying, and somehow to be able to contain and hold these feelings on behalf of the organization.

I shall be considering the role of chaplain when confronted with death and grief in this book, and I will reflect on experiences I have had, particularly in prisons and a hospice. Dealing with death is of course not the only area of chaplaincy ministry, or pastoral care, but it is one which has had a profound impact in my life, and in my ministry, and it is a subject that should be of interest to us all, since we will all have to face death some time.

CHAPTER 2

Understanding Pastoral Care

In this chapter I use experiences from prison and hospice to consider what pastoral care is, both theologically and practically. What are the main components of pastoral relationships? What are the pastoral needs of people who are in prison or who are dying? What are the personal qualities that a pastoral carer needs? What can happen in pastoral relationships?

What is pastoral care?

The consultant in palliative care at our hospice asked me recently what theoretical model I used for the work that I do. It was a question which both intrigued, baffled and challenged me. Most of the time I just get on with doing the job in hand, not really thinking about how I do it. In writing this book I have had to ponder this question more deeply, for I need to be able to understand what pastoral care is and how it happens in order to explain it to others. In my search to answer these questions I have not only returned to books which have remained unopened on my shelves for many years, but I have also reflected on my own experience of pastoral care.

In his book *A Critique of Pastoral Care*, Stephen Pattison quotes a number of descriptions of pastoral care. I feel particularly drawn to this one from *Paid to Care?* by Alastair Campbell:

> Pastoral care is, in essence, surprisingly simple. It has one fundamental aim: to help someone to know love, both as something to be received and as something to give.[1]

Love is the foundation of the Christian gospel message, for we claim that God is Love, and the greatest commandment, Jesus reminds us, from the Jewish tradition, that we should love God with all our heart, mind and strength, and love our neighbour as we love ourselves (see Matthew 22:37).

Pastoral care is one of the ways in which people of faith seek to follow these commandments. For those who come from a secular perspective, and who have been trained in therapeutic disciplines, "love" is probably not a word that appears very frequently. This is possibly where therapy and theology part company.

In engaging with anyone pastorally, my starting point is that they are a child of God, made in God's image and loved by God; that image may be distorted, and they may not believe that they are loved by anyone; they may have no love for themselves; they may have no concept of, or belief in, God. What matters most is not what they believe, but that my beliefs motivate me to have compassion towards them. The Gospels are full of stories of Jesus meeting people who are unloved and excluded; people who have cheated others; people whose physical condition or mental illness kept them imprisoned in their situation and made them outsiders to society. Jesus approached them with love, acceptance and compassion, seeing beyond the limitations of their condition or circumstances or their past, and recognizing their intrinsic value and worth; seeing their qualities and potential; seeing them through the loving eyes of God.

In conversing and listening to people I rarely talk about my theology or faith, but it is what drives me and motivates me to do what I do. I may be with someone who is dying, whose body is emaciated, who has no control over their bodily functions and whose mind is confused; or I may be listening to someone who has caused others great harm and whose self-image is grossly distorted; or I may be with someone who has lost all sense of purpose and meaning and whose only desire is to not exist. In any of these situations as I listen at depth to what they are saying or no longer able to say, and how they present themselves, I am also consciously reminding myself to see them as God sees them; through the eyes of love. For if Campbell's understanding of the aim of pastoral care is correct—to help someone know love—then it is in my engagement with them at that moment that I have the opportunity to show them the meaning of love itself by the way that I relate to them.

My experience of pastoral relationships is that any who are involved may be changed by that encounter, and that each can learn and give something to the other. I have always drawn from the wisdom of the Jewish mystic Martin Buber; he talks of I–Thou connectedness in which God is always present; in which "all real living is meeting".[2] Pastoral care, where there is mutuality, openness, connectedness and where love is expressed, is also spiritual care, for it is engagement at depth with the core of who we are as human beings and with what gives our lives value and meaning.

What are the components of pastoral care?

I have pastorally supported people in many different locations and in life and death circumstances. It has always involved my being open and welcoming, establishing a rapport, building trust and listening attentively. It has been necessary to put aside my own ego, as far as possible, put the other person in the centre and show them unconditional positive regard. Many of the people I have worked amongst have experienced some kind of physical, emotional, sexual or spiritual abuse, so enabling them to feel safe is paramount. My body language, voice, tone and persona will affect how I am perceived—probably even more than the words I may actually say.

There may be multiple components of establishing a safe pastoral therapeutic relationship. I wish to highlight seven which I have found to be essential. These are:

1. Attentiveness
2. Active listening
3. Accompaniment
4. Authenticity
5. Compassion
6. Containment
7. Challenge

Attentiveness

Being attentive requires the pastor to be comfortable enough in themselves not to impose themselves on the other person, and to be open to the encounter between them. The phrase "getting oneself out of the way" seems fitting. Attentiveness means being fully present in that moment—not allowing the concerns about a later meeting, or unfinished business waiting to be done, to dominate one's thoughts. It can be hard work to be attentive.

Sometimes it can be helpful to all those involved to lay out the time available for the encounter. If you only have thirty minutes available at that moment, then it is fine to say so; it gives the person being listened to a boundary, and it avoids the feelings of frustration or even panic that the listener may feel if the conversation seems to be running on and on.

I have noticed on many occasions when a conversation has been time-bound, the most pressing concern or question is only expressed towards the end of the encounter. I first experienced this in my time as a speech therapist. I called this "the door handle remark". Often the client raised this matter at the end of the time for a particular reason—conscious or unconscious—and respecting that reason was part of being attentive. It was important to acknowledge the enormity of the issue raised, to recognize that it was not possible to do it justice in the time remaining, but that it would be followed up on another occasion if appropriate.

Active listening

At the heart of all pastoral relationships is the ability to listen. Most of us think we can listen, and probably take it for granted that we do. However, the quality of our listening as well as the depth of how we are listened to varies considerably.

Gerard Hughes SJ sums it up:

> The gift of being a good listener, a gift which requires constant practice, is perhaps the most healing gift anyone can possess, for it allows the other to be, enfolds them in a safe place, does not judge or advise them, accepts them as they are without desiring to change them, and communicates support at a level deeper than words.[3]

Active listening involves the listener reflecting back to the speaker what they have heard; it is hearing not only what is said, but what is not said; picking up and reading the signs of someone's mental, emotional, psychological and spiritual state; knowing when to stay, and when to leave; recognizing the time to speak and the time to remain silent, and being comfortable in silence, which can speak volumes.

Accompaniment

Accompanying someone as they journey means walking alongside them, at their pace, and in the direction they choose. In music, accompaniment is the instrument or part which is played at the same time as a soloist, supporting the melody and forming the background to it. In the hospice our music therapist sees patients on the ward. He takes a trolley of instruments into the patient's room. The patient improvises with an instrument or in song, and the therapist follows and supports them by his accompaniment on the keyboard. The patient is frequently surprised by the quality of music created together. The pastor, similarly, accompanies people; going at their pace, following their lead, not dominating, but responding. There are rises and falls in the music or encounter, different keys, styles and tempos. The accompaniment by the pastor sustains and supports the conversation and the outcome can surprise and delight all the participants.

Authenticity

In any pastoral encounter being true to oneself and genuine in one's responses is essential. If there is the slightest hint of being formulaic in my responses or if I appear to wear a mask of "professional" in a pastoral encounter, the conversation will remain superficial. People who are at a point of great need and who are vulnerable because they are in prison, or are dying, will detect insincerity straight away. As a pastor in training in my curacy, I worked with people who were homeless, and found that they were less inhibited by social niceties than others; for some, alcohol contributed to their being forthright. They would tell you outright if they perceived that they were being fobbed off or patronized or that you were not genuine. I am grateful to these people for their honesty which helped my development as a pastoral carer enormously. Perhaps it should be a compulsory part of ministerial formation to work in this sort of setting? In other contexts, perhaps, people are more guarded about saying what they think, especially to someone with perceived authority such as a priest or minister. Meaningful encounters with someone in distress or need will happen when the pastor is honest, real, and allows themselves to be vulnerable in doing so.

Compassion

This is an area which some might say differs depending on the context. How can you have compassion, some would argue, for a murderer, a rapist, a paedophile? Surely they are getting what they deserve, and not a moment too soon! It is not my role or position or intention to judge those in my care. I look for the humanity in someone. Compassion goes beyond just being non-judgemental, which is a passive response and avoids looking at the darker side of the person for fear of what it may generate within us. Compassion is active; it recognizes the wholeness of the individual, sees them warts and all, sees the burdens they may carry, of guilt and shame, and reaches out to them. Compassion is associated with warmth, love, kindness and help. In a pastoral situation it is a way of recognizing that by being with another person I am offering them something, being supportive, and that in doing so I am making a difference.

In the Gospels, Jesus is often described as having compassion. His presence offers healing to those who are distressed, but he sees them in every dimension and facet.

There is a difference between compassion and empathy and these feelings are elicited from different areas of the brain. Empathy is the emotional response when one places oneself in the shoes of another person. It is generally associated with feelings of sadness. On the ward in a hospice often there is a huge amount of sadness; as patients and their families face the prospect of loss and permanent separation. The staff who move from one room to the next constantly have to manage their own feelings in response to the pain of others. If someone is very empathetic to each patient, then they will soon become overwhelmed by their own emotions and are likely to get burned out. It is possible to switch between compassion and empathy constantly and in a challenging pastoral encounter this can be extremely helpful. Understanding our own emotional responses and reflecting on them away from the immediately painful situation can also help to develop emotional and spiritual resilience.

I discovered the cost of empathy when I was a young speech therapist. I worked in a very deprived area of East London, with many families living in poverty. Many were refugees and had come from complex situations. As I listened to their experiences and saw their living conditions I empathized with them; as I put myself in their position I became overwhelmed with pain and sadness, and I felt impotent to do anything about it. Offering support for their child's speech and language deficit seemed only to scratch the surface of their needs. It made me feel overwhelmed and ultimately led to my own experience of depression.

In Holloway Prison young women who were facing lengthy sentences, or whose lifestyles were destructive, sometimes had to face giving their children up for adoption. As chaplain, I supported several women through this process. At the time I was a mother of young children myself; if I empathized too much with the woman's situation, and placed myself in her shoes, I could easily have become overwhelmed. I had to work hard to tell myself that this painful experience was not mine; the sadness I felt was mostly coming from the woman herself. I had to tell myself that by listening, or accompanying the woman on her last visit with her child, I was being a help and support to her. I was moving between empathy and compassion in this encounter and in doing so was able to offer more support to the woman.

Containment

If people are going to share with me the depths of their need and pain, they need not only to trust me, though that is essential, but they also need to trust that I will not get overwhelmed by what they are sharing. If someone feels that the person they are talking to cannot hold what they are telling them, they will either not discuss all that they need to, or they will reverse the roles and start offering care to the pastor. While there is mutuality in the exchange, and both will be changed by the encounter, this is not the time for the pastor to get psychological support from the person who has come to talk to them. Containment is holding with integrity what is being shared. It is more than confidentiality, which is also essential for building up trust—it is being able to provide a place of psychological safety for difficult and painful things to be named, considered and left behind.

Challenge

As I reread Stephen Pattison's book *A Critique of Pastoral Care*, I was struck by his insistence that pastoral care contains challenge. Initially I resisted this concept as it felt too harsh, possibly hierarchical, and confrontational. However, I have considered the many situations I have been in, and can see that if trust is established and the components I have described above are present, then challenge has often been a creative part of pastoral situations. The manner in which a challenge is made must be taken into consideration; also, the pastor must be clear why they need to be challenging. Pastoral care is not about solving other people's problems or giving advice. If pastoral care is about knowing love, then in some circumstances challenging someone can be the most loving response, enabling greater growth and personal development than would be achieved if one was simply showing empathy. Challenges can only be made when a relationship of mutual respect and acceptance is in place.

I spoke to a young woman, Chloe, who had just arrived in Downview Prison. Her reputation as a difficult and disruptive person had preceded her. She had been so hard to manage in other prisons that she was being moved around every few weeks to give the staff a break. When she arrived, I went to see her as part of my chaplaincy duties. She began to be mouthy and unpleasant, so I put it to her that she had a choice—she could continue to behave in the same way wherever she went, get everyone's back up and waste her time, or she could look at this as a fresh start and use the opportunities that being in prison afforded—to get an education or learn a skill. She had probably been told this by uniformed staff on many occasions, but perhaps the fact that I was a chaplain whom she had not expected to be so forthright had greater effect. We went on to build a relationship of immense trust and goodwill, and her attitude changed dramatically.

What are the pastoral needs of prisoners or those who are dying?

Dame Cicely Saunders, founder of the modern hospice movement, talked of "total pain"—suffering at many levels—in her work with people who are dying. There is physical pain, which should be alleviated wherever possible with medication; social pain, the loss of company, friendship and lifestyle as circumstances change with illness; emotional pain as people experience strong feelings of fear, anger, sorrow, despair and anxiety; and spiritual pain which includes questions of worth, value, meaning, as well as matters related to faith and God. Why is God letting this happen to me? Where is God now? How can a good person deserve this suffering?

Having come across the notion of total pain in the hospice movement I have reflected back on my ministry in prisons, and see that it could be applied to the experience of prisoners. There are physical pains of being in prison—the harshness of the environment; the loss of privacy; being strip-searched; sharing a small room with strangers; the locked doors; jangling keys; the noise. People who come to prison for the first time are often in shock, numbed by the initial experience, and can feel physically sick and distressed at the concern for their families, especially their children—women in particular feel this pain acutely. Prisoners who are detoxing from drugs or alcohol experience excruciating physical symptoms of pain, sweats, shaking, nausea and sleep deprivation. The social pains of imprisonment are clear, separation from family being one. Prisons by their very nature are closed environments designed to separate the general public from criminals. People in prison feel like social pariahs and may be treated as such by family, friends and society, whilst they are in prison, or on their release. They may lose their jobs, their home, their money, their prospects. The emotional pains of being in prison are often depression, despair, lethargy, apathy, despondency, grief. Prisoners may feel that they are no longer people, that they are a number only; they may feel that they no longer know who they are any more, that they will be labelled simply as criminal, and no one will ever be able to see them as anything other than this. They lose all hope. These are spiritual pains.

I encountered enormous numbers of people experiencing emotional and spiritual pain in prison. Prisoners carry with them huge amounts of baggage from their past, things they have done, as well as things that have been done to them. Coming to prison may be the first time that they have actually had time and space to reflect on themselves, and that is not always comfortable. There will be some, of course, who don't want to think about these things, and will spend their time in prison continuing their chaotic lives and searching for ways to do so, through continued addictions, use of prescribed medication, or their behaviours towards others. There may be others who do not want help, they may be so despondent and despairing that there seems no point in living as they are simply existing, and they might as well be dead.

As a chaplain my primary concern is not with retribution and justice, but with mercy and love. I believe that people are changed internally not by intimidation, but by recognizing their worth and value, though sometimes it is buried deep within. I used to have on my desk in the prison a postcard from the Quaker Tapestry. It has shaped my way of thinking about prisoners and my ministry within prisons in addressing their spiritual pains:

> Quakers believe that there is that of God in all people, though it is sometimes hard to find. Punishment ought to be a way of helping people realize the hurt they are doing to this sense of worth in themselves and in others.[4]

When people are dying, like people in prison they may look back at their lives reflectively. There may be regret for missed opportunities, or for things they wished they had done differently. There may be sadness about relationships that have been broken and not been repaired. There may be anger and bitterness about previous life experiences; this anger is buried deep but can resurface. It is the dramatic changes of circumstance—facing death or imprisonment—that can prompt soul-searching which can be uncomfortable or distressing. In the hospice, this can become apparent when no amount of medication seems to alleviate the patient's symptoms of pain, and when this happens the multi-disciplinary team considers offering other forms of psychological and spiritual support. Sometimes it is a healthcare assistant or a volunteer who is taking in the tea who will hear the patient's distress and act as a confessor; sometimes it will be the consultant or the housekeeper. Everyone in the hospice needs to be open and ready to hear and respond to pain of any kind.

What personal qualities does a pastoral carer need?

Caring for people pastorally could be described as an art or a skill, and it requires practice. There may be some whose personality and approach to life are better suited to this kind of work than others. A pastoral carer has to be open to the possibility of change in themselves as well as in the other person. And they must hold on to the belief that change can occur, without presuming to anticipate how or in what way change may happen; in this sense they are a bearer of hope.

A pastoral carer is not a problem-solver, or a giver of advice. They are more like a mirror, reflecting back to the speaker what they are hearing. This ability to reframe what someone else says can be remarkably helpful; it can enable the speaker to hear themselves in a different way and may help them to shift perspective and perceptions. A pastor can also reflect back feelings that they observe in the tone and demeanour of the speaker, or that they identify in themselves through transference; for those who find identifying emotions or talking about them difficult, this can be enlightening. If what is reflected back is not what the speaker is trying to say, or not what they feel exactly, then this can also be valuable, because the speaker can say:

> It's not that I feel sad, but actually I feel really angry about my situation.

A pastor should be emotionally articulate and literate to be able to converse at this level with others.

In order to listen and reflect back to others it is imperative that the pastor is self-aware and reflective themselves. It is helpful for a pastor to understand and recognize the drama triangle of rescuer, persecutor and victim, which was developed by Stephen Karpman in 1968, as part of the transactional analysis of relationships. It is important to avoid slipping into these roles as a pastoral carer. Another triangle, the winners' triangle, replaces rescuer with nurturer; persecutor with assertive; and victim with vulnerable. A nurturer is a person who shows understanding and gives care when asked but does not need to be needed; the one who is assertive knows their own feelings and can name them, and speaks using the first person—"I feel", "I think"; and the person who is vulnerable is not weak, but recognizes their limitations, accepts themselves as they are and is able to be authentic and real.

As a pastoral carer one must carry a degree of self-confidence and assurance; this is not assuming certainty or being arrogant or self-righteous but is being humble and patient and using wisdom acquired through one's own struggles with pain at many levels. A pastor is not a counsellor, so is not bound to the structures of engagement in the same way; nevertheless, having boundaries of space, time and availability are important if a pastor is going to continue in this kind of in-depth support of others for any length of time.

I have encountered many people who are extremely complicated at an emotional, social and spiritual level; who are demanding of vast amounts of time and energy. There are people whom no amount of support or care seems to satisfy. I have developed a short-hand term for people who are like this as "needy, greedy". It is psychologically fatal to try and rescue or problem-solve such people. In some circumstances it may be that all a pastoral carer can do is to be assertive, to try to see these challenging people in a loving way as God sees them, and to hand them over spiritually into God's care.

What can happen in a pastoral encounter?

Because every situation and every individual is different, there is no single thing that will happen in a pastoral encounter. I spend so much of my life listening to others that I can easily forget that many people have very limited opportunities to be listened to and to voice their thoughts, fears and emotions. Instead they carry the weight of their concerns around, and may ruminate on them for days, weeks or even years. Dwelling on the same issues and not being able to see a way forward in dealing with them, or not being able to tell someone what one really feels, can lead to many kinds of mental ill health and distress. So the very fact of being able to say something out loud can be healing in itself. Often people describe a weight being lifted, or feeling lighter at the end of the conversation, and it can be apparent in their body language and presentation that this is the case.

People in prison have a great deal of time to dwell on their lives and situations. They may not trust other prisoners enough to talk to them openly; they will generally be guarded. They may resist speaking to an officer for fear of how information about them will be used; they may have a general mistrust of figures in authority. If they have any family that they can talk to it will be in a visiting room packed with other people, and if they talk on the phone, it will be in a public place where they will be observed and overheard, and calls may be monitored for security purposes. Prisoners may not want to talk to their family or may find it hard to be honest with them about how they are feeling. In the same way, people who are dying may be reticent about speaking to their families—they don't want to worry or burden them further. Families—both of prisoners and people who are dying—may also find it hard to talk openly to their relative. An impartial pastoral carer who listens may be very welcome in these circumstances.

Often when someone is listened to in a pastoral conversation, their perspective on their situation or themselves alters. It is as if, by hearing themselves articulate their thoughts and struggles with something, they begin to view things in a new light. Sometimes at the start of a conversation people say that they are not very good at expressing themselves, or that they find trusting people difficult. At the end of the encounter I may gently point out to them that they have now been able to talk and trust me. Sometimes I ask them to reflect on their feelings when they first came into the room, and how they are feeling at the end of the conversation; I may ask them to identify their feelings on a numbered scale. Frequently people notice a positive change, even a small one, and begin to recognize the value of talking and being heard. This may lead me to suggest they could look for support from other people, agencies or therapists, because if they have found they can open up to me, then they may be able to do so with others.

When people have described difficult life experiences or when they feel they have made errors of judgement and wrong choices, I invite them to consider what they have learned from these situations. I have frequently said to people that no experience is wasted if we can learn from it. This prompts them to go beyond self-recrimination and self-loathing, which takes them nowhere, and to become more reflective and hopeful about themselves. Reminding people that they cannot change the choices that they have made, but they can try and make different choices in the future, can also enable them to see that mistakes are not necessarily disastrous, but that they can be opportunities for growth and development.

Pastoral care can help someone who has opened up in conversation to feel less isolated. They have shared something that matters to them, and which they may have felt shame or regret about. They may feel that they have been able to connect in a meaningful way, because someone has listened to them carefully and without judgement. People who have been bereaved, for example, often feel that they are going mad, because they are not able to function in the way that they did before their loss. If I can reflect back to them that the feelings they are describing are part of the uncomfortable reality of grief, and that others in similar situations have expressed similar feelings, then they may feel less worried about their own reactions.

People who have struggles with addictions, and who want to change, can be particularly hard on themselves when they have a relapse. In my experience it is not uncommon to meet people who have been in and out of prison because of drug-related offences. They can easily become despairing of themselves and want to give up trying. It is so important as a pastoral carer never to give up on anyone and to continue to hold the belief in the possibility that people can change. Sometimes it is hard to break through that despondency and despair, but telling them that they are a person of worth no matter how many falls they have had, and that people sometimes go round and around the system of drugs and prison before they finally break free, can give them something to cling on to. I have said many times to people who are struggling that even if they cannot see hope for themselves, I am holding the candle of hope for them.

For many people forgiveness of themselves as well as forgiveness of others is part of the journey towards healing. I spent some time talking to a woman whose husband was dying. She carried a great deal of anger. As we talked it became apparent that the anger she felt was not because her husband was dying, but because of how he had been for much of their married life. Now that he was close to death, she felt immense guilt that she had felt negatively towards him, especially when he had been so unwell. In my presence she was able to recognize and acknowledge her real feelings; we then explored the possibility of her talking openly to her husband in his final days. I saw her a few days later. The anger she had been expressing previously was replaced with sadness at her husband's impending death. She had been able to be honest with her husband, and they had recognized fault on both sides, and had made their peace with one another. They had both acknowledged wrong and forgiven each other. He then was able to die peacefully and her grief would not be further complicated by regret, guilt and remorse.

Sometimes it is when someone recognizes what unforgiveness looks like that they decide that they want to let go of the inner rage and turmoil that they are carrying around. It has been revelatory to many people to recognize that their anger has no impact on the person who has hurt them. Forgiveness cannot be imposed on others or forced as a requirement. I have found that hearing or reading about others who have forgiven can help another person make a shift in themselves to do so. Forgiving oneself can be even more difficult.

People I have encountered pastorally have changed in many ways; they may have let go of hurts; recognized that they are not alone in their struggle; learned to live with their past; found some purpose in their present experiences; accepted a situation which cannot be changed; or found peace. Celebrating with people their developments in self-awareness, self-acceptance and new experiences has been a delight and privilege. I discovered a new phrase recently which I shall add to my armoury of pastoral insights: post-traumatic growth. It seems a wonderful tool to support people as they struggle to make sense of their experiences of pain and suffering.

Of course, not everyone who engages with pastoral care is able to change or grow and as a pastoral carer I have had to accept this on many occasions. Pastoral care is never offered in a vacuum; and it is not about fulfilling my needs and making myself feel positive about what I do.

People change at different rates and in different circumstances. I may not be the one to see someone move on, but someone else who supports that person at another time in their life may. I hope that if nothing else I have been able to make a meaningful connection with someone; have given them a good experience of being listened to, heard or accompanied; and have demonstrated in my engagement with them that they are a person of worth.

I visited a residential care home for people with advanced dementia. The residents were mostly incapable of speaking; many were nursed in bed. Pastoral care in this situation was clearly not going to be at the level of listening and verbal communication and there was going to be no change in their outlook or circumstance. However, by being fully present in the moment with each resident, by holding their hand, by talking quietly and gently to them or by holding their gaze I hope I was communicating that I saw them as a person of value. I was making a connection with them at a deep level of compassion, love and shared humanity. Their brokenness in body and mind caused me to think again about the meaning of personhood, challenged me to see them as God sees them, caused me to reflect theologically on the image of the Body of Christ, and drew from me immense compassion and empathy. In this pastoral situation, as in so many others, the residents I met became my teachers, and I was the one who experienced profound change.

Pastoral encounters

Adam

On introducing myself to one patient, Adam, as he played Scrabble with one of the healthcare assistants, his immediate response on seeing me was to state clearly that he was an atheist. My response to him was:

> That's great! We can have some interesting conversations then, if you like?

In a hospice you may have little time or opportunity to establish a rapport and relationship. I said hello in passing a few times, and after a while he invited me to sit down in his room whilst he ate his lunch. On one occasion I collected my own sandwiches, and we ate together. We had a fascinating conversation about his interests in history, his enthusiasm for model-making and his knowledge as an engineer. Over time our conversations broadened to his motivations in life, his family relations, his love of music. All of these elements contributed to my fuller understanding of Adam as a person, what makes him tick and the essence of who he is. I hope I reassured Adam that I had no other agenda than to be interested in him as a fellow human being.

Adam had spent much of his life alienating people by his criticisms of them; he held most people at arm's length and was lacking in skill and confidence in making meaningful relationships. Adam spent the last few weeks of his life in the hospice. One of Cicely Saunders' most well-known statements about the work of the hospice movement is this:

> You matter because you are you, and you matter until the moment you die. We will do all that we can to help you die peacefully and to live until you die.

I believe that the care the hospice staff gave to Adam demonstrated this clearly. Adam was treated with acceptance, humour and compassion; he learned to give and receive kindness; he learned more about the goodness of humanity than he had ever experienced before. Though his body diminished as a result of his cancer, his spirit flourished and he became a much wiser and more caring person than ever before. I was able to share this observation with a relative who organized his burial which I and a colleague from the hospice attended. Though to society Adam's life may have had little to show for it, his dying and death was very gracious and meaningful and loving. As he was closer to death, I shared with him all that I had valued in the few weeks I had known him. I thanked him for his friendship and, careful not to impose my beliefs on him, I said, "Bless you, Adam," and his response to me was, "Bless *you*." Adam taught all of us a great deal. He would be very tickled, I am sure, that I would be including him in this book. Through establishing a meaningful engagement with Adam, or any others that I encounter, I hope to reawaken their sense of self-worth and value, at a time when they can otherwise feel hopeless and useless.

Terry

I met one prisoner, Terry, soon after I came to the Isle of Wight; looking back now I see that he was experiencing total pain. His self-esteem was so low that he could barely look me in the eye when I talked to him. He found it impossible to call me anything other than Miss; eventually he told me that to call me by my name suggested a connection which he felt completely unworthy of making. He loathed himself so much that despite his boots leaking, and his feet rotting in them, he preferred to be in physical pain than to ask for new ones. He had been in prison for nearly twenty years, and in this one for a decade. He refused to engage with any rehabilitation programmes, because that would mean he would progress in the prison system, which he did not want to do. He wanted to die in prison, this Category B prison, as this was all he deserved. He was a very driven man, however, and spent hours running on the sports ground, pushing himself in an extreme way. I don't know whether this helped to clear his mind from his torment, or whether it caused him additional physical pain. He had cut off all ties with his family. He said he was the one who deserved to come to prison, he didn't want his family to have to endure visits or any contact.

Terry was so hardened that he refused to show any emotion, even when telling me of multiple bereavements he had experienced as a child, but I felt his pain. I took some comfort from the fact that he would at least talk to me. In fact, I sometimes stood for lengthy periods, in all weathers, listening to him, as his job, at which he excelled, was as a gardener. Generally, I would end conversations with male prisoners by shaking their hand, as a gesture of humanity. I offered to shake Terry's hand after one conversation. He responded by saying that he never allowed anyone to touch him, because it would make a human connection which he did not feel worthy of. He described himself as "scum", a "nobody", and he really believed it. He could not accept or even hear another narrative which I sometimes described to him, the Christian message of love and forgiveness. He was in a place of such darkness of self-disgust, that it seemed no light or love could penetrate it.

I came away from our conversations greatly saddened by Terry's total absence of hope and purpose, and his inability to see himself in any positive light. Indeed, he had lived with this way of thinking about himself for so long, that to contemplate change seemed like a betrayal of years of his existence. I felt frustrated that the prison system had reinforced his self-hatred, and could do nothing to rehabilitate this man, who was a similar age to myself, and could live for another thirty years in the same stuck place.

However, my lack of faith was challenged immensely when he told me one day that he had begun to read *The Shack*, by William P. Young. I had been leading a weekly study group on this book with some of the prisoners. One had lent Terry the book. This book, and the subsequent conversations he must have had on the wing with this prisoner, transformed Terry. It was little short of miraculous. Having heard him say many times that he had never been in a church and would never go in one, because he was so unworthy, I was bowled over to see him in chapel on Palm Sunday. In fact, I didn't recognize him at first, without his cap and overalls on, wearing his prison-issue striped shirt and jeans. He came to all the services of Holy Week that year, including the Maundy Thursday foot-washing in which he took part by allowing me to wash his hands. He came to the chapel for several weeks, though he said that he felt so choked that he couldn't utter a single sound. He went on to make contact again with his family; he accepted progression out of a Category B prison and left to continue his sentence.

Tina

A nurse had identified that a patient was experiencing spiritual and emotional pain, and I was asked to visit her. I found a small, frail woman, who was in her late sixties but looked considerably older. She was curled over in her chair and barely able to hold her head up or make eye contact. She peppered her conversation with apologies and repeatedly said that she was not making much sense. I reassured her that what she was expressing was quite understandable. Here was an educated woman, Tina, who was lost, frightened, and angry at her situation. She felt cheated that she was not going to enjoy a long retirement, as she had expected to do, and she was horrified at having to be so dependent on others. She described herself as feeling hemmed in, imprisoned by her condition within four walls, and she had no idea who she was any more. I asked her what mattered most to her at the moment; she said, "Getting better. Getting rid of this illness."

She knew that this was not possible, as her condition was terminal.

I felt Tina was expressing physical, emotional, social and spiritual pain in her demeanour as well as in her conversation. I shared with her the idea of total pain, and she responded warmly to this notion, recognizing that there were pains at much deeper levels that were causing her distress. She talked about the changes that were happening in her relationship and the strain it was causing to her and her partner. She loathed the loss of dignity she felt when others had to take care of her very personal needs. She was enraged, though she was unable to use this language herself. By listening, and by reflecting back to her what she was expressing, I acted like a mirror to her thoughts and feelings. I gave her permission to feel the strong emotions which she hinted at, and reassured her that these were human responses to immensely challenging changes of circumstance. We talked about her grief. I told her of Cicely Saunders' vision of care for the dying—that you matter because you are you—and affirmed her in her intrinsic worth and value as a human being whatever her physical condition. As I left she was sitting more upright in her chair, her head held higher, and looked me in the eye. She looked younger. I asked her again what mattered most to her. She replied, "Finding peace."

Tina continued to struggle with her situation, and after the ward round the following week the consultant asked me to see her, as he felt that her pain was less physical and more spiritual. It was Maundy Thursday. I listened again to Tina's pain and her anger. I described a scene from the film *The Mission*, in which a tortured individual tries to pull a sword up a steep ravine as penance for wrongs he has done in his life. It is only when the rope holding the load is cut away that he is free. I suggested to Tina that she was carrying around a heavy boulder and that only she could let it go. I saw Tina again on Easter Day. She came to the chapel service with her husband and received Communion. I read the story of Mary Magdalene in the garden and invited comments, as is my custom, from those who were gathered. Tina spoke very movingly about her feelings.

When I spoke to nursing staff later, they said that Tina had returned from the service looking different.

I went to see her. She told me that she had had a light bulb moment after our conversation on Maundy Thursday. It had clearly been a soul-searching and emotional experience. She had come to see that she had been feeling angry and that this was getting in the way of everything else, affecting her relationship with her husband and spoiling the short amount of time they might have left together. She was critical of herself for letting it happen like this, but she was now perfectly clear that she didn't feel angry any longer. She was able to say, what will be will be, I cannot change it, but I want to make the best of the time that I have left. She described feeling better—though there was no change in her cancer. It was a momentous transformation, which was quite inspirational to see. I told her that I wished I could bottle this experience and pass it on to others, but that in reality each individual has to find their own way through. However, I told her that I was writing this book, and she was delighted to think that her experience might help someone else. It gave an additional purpose to her suffering.

Tina had found the peace for which she was searching. She looked, sounded and talked very differently now to when I had first seen her. She no longer said sorry constantly; she no longer questioned whether she was making sense or commented that what she said was stupid. She was self-assured, confident and dignified. She had rediscovered her sense of self, and with that came a strength which perhaps she had never felt before. She said of herself, I feel resilient. I asked her if there was any change in her husband, and she felt there was. It seemed that as she showed an ability to cope with her situation, so he was able to relax too, and let go of some of his anger. I commented that this was a wonderful legacy to leave him, passing on her strength to him.

There is no doubt in my mind that Tina had changed; perhaps this was her life's work. In our final conversation in the hospice, I thanked Tina for her openness, her honesty, and for all that she had taught me by allowing me to share this part of her life with her. I learned from her so much: about spiritual distress and pain; about never losing hope or faith, even in the face of death; in the power of love to transform and heal at a level way beyond the physical; that resurrection happens. It is not always the length of our encounters that matters, but the depths which are explored within them. All this took place within ten days covering the whole of the Passion, Holy Week and Easter Day. Tina was preparing to go home. The equipment was in place and the transfer was due to take place as soon as transport was arranged. However, she died sooner than was expected, the day after this conversation.

I return to the initial question which began this chapter: what is the theoretical model of pastoral care? In considering this I have identified that pastoral care does not have a single model as a starting point, but it begins from a theological perspective of love and acceptance. Therapy is generally a contractual agreement of time and frequency, and operates from a particular theoretical model of care, such as Jungian or person-centred. Pastoral care may draw on these perspectives but is not defined by them. Pastoral encounters are often spontaneous, can be limited to a single conversation and may last for anything from a few minutes to several hours. Pastoral care cannot be measured in outcomes or outputs, though some would like it to be. It is an organic, relational process; using the language of theology, it is guided and shaped by the Holy Spirit. Pastoral care differs from person to person, depending on the gifts and self-awareness of the people involved. It requires a willingness to become vulnerable to one another, to risk being challenged and changed by the encounter, and the awareness that each can learn and grow as the conversation and relationship develops. Fundamental to all pastoral encounters is the ability to listen, without judgement, and holding on to the hope and belief that healing and transformation can happen when a person is helped to know how to receive and give love.

CHAPTER 3

Dying Well

Having looked at my own experience of chaplaincy in various contexts, and at the foundation of all chaplaincy work which is pastoral care, in the following chapters I consider the specific pastoral matter of death and dying. In this chapter I reflect on how death is understood and faced in modern Western society. I describe a good death from a religious and non-religious perspective. I draw on personal experiences of such deaths, including the death of my father.

In this technological age and in the Western developed world there are machines to take on many menial tasks, and science and engineering advances create the impression that humanity is invincible. Humanity is more able to control its environment than ever before. However, the art of dying has not been mastered, and no technology or advancement of science has yet found the way to prevent it happening. Cryo-preservation comes the closest to avoiding death by freezing the bodies of those who have died in the hope that technology will advance to such an extent that they can be revived in a later generation. This would create ethical and practical dilemmas should it ever be realized and available to more than those with a vast income. Mitch Albom considers these matters in his novel, *The Timekeeper*. Perhaps one day the formula for immortality will be discovered, but that in itself would generate a whole host of other problems for the human race and the environment. It is questionable whether such a discovery would be progress at all. Until such an "advance" is made, then, society and individuals must face, wrestle with, learn from and experience the reality of death. The sooner we can do so with maturity, humour, acceptance and honesty, the healthier we will become emotionally, physically and spiritually.

As an Anglican priest, death and dying is something which I have had to think about. Before being ordained and even when I was going through the training to be a priest, I felt really concerned and anxious about having to deal with death. I was always a very emotional child: I cried at every remotely sad film and was very sensitive to any situation of human tragedy. I also had a very great fear of losing someone close to me. The thought of being a priest where I would be expected to be able to hold things together emotionally when facing someone who was dying or when taking a funeral was unimaginable.

I have had to face those fears. Since being ordained in 1996 I have had the experience of being with those who are dying in a variety of situations. It has been an experience which I have found deeply enriching, humbling and life changing for me. I realize, however, that many people will have very little opportunity of being alongside dying people, except those that they are especially close to, or indeed when they face their own death. I hope that by sharing my experiences and reflections I can help those who read this to face their own or another's death.

I am indebted to those people who have permitted me to share their final hours and who have invited me to accompany them through their experience of dying. Each one has taught me so much; shared so much; entrusted so much. In telling the stories of people's dying, I seek not to dishonour or breach the trust that has been placed in me, but to voice what they cannot, to describe what no one else can.

I write as a Christian who believes that death is not the extinguishing of life, but the gate through which we must all pass. I have no definite description of what lies beyond death, though I have some hopes about it. I make no attempt to impose my beliefs onto others. I hope what I write here will interest those of any faith perspective and none, for death is universal—it is what unites the whole of humanity when so much else divides us. Dying and death will have to be faced by each of us sometime. I just hope that whoever reads this now will face this inevitability with less fear and more courage, knowing that others have travelled this way before.

A good death

In traditional Roman Catholicism a good death is defined as having confessed one's sins before God, been absolved by the priest, and received the sacrament of Holy Communion. The dying person will then be in a state of grace, and not in a state of mortal sin, ready to go right to heaven. On the other hand, the Institute of Medicine defines a good death as

> one that is free from avoidable distress and suffering, for patients, family, and caregivers; in general accord with the patients' and families' wishes; and reasonably consistent with clinical, cultural, and ethical standards.

One of the very few sermons I remember from my time at theological college was by my vicar from London, who had come to Cambridge to preach at our evening service. She recounted the recent death of a parishioner with whom I was acquainted. It was during this sermon that I heard for the first time the term, "a good death". It was a phrase which has stayed with me throughout my ministry and is something which I have now had experience of myself.

A good death, as I now understand it, is one where the dying person is prepared and ready to go; maybe they have been able to say their farewells to loved ones, perhaps the loved ones are actually present at the moment of death. The person dying is in as little physical pain as possible; is either in their own home or in comfortable surroundings; and just slips away, after a long and fulfilling life. When I was pregnant, I was encouraged to write a birth plan for the arrival of each of my three children. If we were each encouraged to write a "death plan", I guess many of us would include many of the aspects of dying well which I have described.

As one who has accompanied people at this moment of their lives, I see a similarity with the role of midwife. At both ends of life, there is a role for one to be alongside, supporting, waiting, encouraging and reassuring. A midwife will have had many experiences of birth, in a way the mother-to-be cannot possibly have had. A priest, or a palliative care nurse who is a companion of someone who is dying, is likely to have had more experience of dying than the person who is experiencing it, or their relatives. Even if it is the first time of being in this situation, somehow the role you have at that moment can in itself be reassuring.

Pastoral encounters

I vividly recall the first death at which I was present. A wonderful woman, Sally, from our congregation, was dying at home, and her children had contacted the local church to ask if someone could come and say prayers with them. I was a curate, in my very early days of ministry, and my vicar suggested that I should go with him for the experience. I was nervous. Here was the first of the hurdles I had to overcome to ensure I was capable of being professional and not too emotional. I had no idea how I would react, or what I would encounter in the situation or in myself.

I know Sally would have been very happy to have had me there as a novice in this position. She had welcomed me with open arms when I came to the church a few months previously. She had watched me learn the roles of leading worship, heard my faltering first sermons and seen me preside at the Eucharist. She was an encourager, a teacher, a fellow believer and a mature friend. I don't think we had ever had the opportunity to talk specifically about her death and dying, but I know for certain that it was not something she was afraid of; her only fear, as is so often the case, was for her children and how they would be without her.

I had never met Sally's children previously, but they were so welcoming and grateful that we were coming to the house to share this experience with them. It can be quite lonely and frightening for those sitting alongside someone in their final hours, especially when verbal communication has ceased and the dying person is no longer responsive. Often people don't know how to be; should they continue to talk to their relative? Should they move? Could they leave the room, and what would happen if the person died when they weren't there? Was it OK to drink tea, or even to laugh? Would they know when the person had actually died, what did this look like? People can feel very disempowered in this situation, understandably so, for it is one they have only experienced occasionally, if at all, and it is generally a time of great emotional turmoil.

A priest or minister can be a reassuring presence. They can say some words of comfort from the Bible, or some familiar prayers, which helps the family, as well as the dying person. Before the dying person becomes unresponsive, the last rites may include receiving the sacrament of Holy Communion. In some traditions, oil which has been blessed can be used to anoint the person on the forehead, hands and sometimes feet, as a symbolic way of preparing them for the next journey. It may be helpful to the family gathered to anoint the dying person too, as a sign of their acceptance of the process of letting them go and blessing them on their way. These gestures and actions can give those who are feeling helpless the sense that they are doing something meaningful. They are often the moments when barriers of pain and sorrow are unleashed, and there is an internal shift for everyone, including the dying person, I believe. These are frequently the most profound and touching experiences, when whoever is present bonds and connects together in an encounter which transcends time and space.

In Sally's situation we said prayers, read psalms and anointed her with oil. Dying is not a science, and although you may know someone is close to the end of their life, you can never know when the moment of death will come. In the same way as waiting for a birth, where there are signs and signals that the arrival is imminent, so with dying, there are different phases of breath to show that the time of the final breath is drawing nearer. But there is a lot of waiting. As a companion, one may become mesmerized by the rhythm of breath, the gentle rise and fall of the chest, or the agonizing rattle of dying, which is so painful to witness.

Monty was one of the first prisoners I journeyed with to his death. He was a very intelligent and thoughtful person, who loved to talk. We built up a good rapport over the months of his declining health and had some very stimulating conversations about whether people would ever acquire the ability to become immortal. Even though he thought it would happen one day, it was clear that it never was going to in time for him! It was before the days of palliative care beds in our prison, so he was taken to the local hospice to die. (I never imagined that years later I would work in this very establishment as chaplain myself!) His parents were very elderly and unable to visit him, and he had no contact with his adult children. He valued the company which I gave him and requested that I should be with him when he died, if possible. As a chaplain there are occasions when one is on call. I kept the phone by my bed and was awoken with the request to come to the hospice, as it seemed that Monty would not last much longer. I arrived at the hospice and came to sit with Monty and the officer who was with him. I sat for a long time, said some prayers and chatted to the member of staff, an experienced officer who had been in this situation before. I was quite new to this role, and wondered how long we would wait, and whether I should remain here until the very end. Monty was unresponsive, and his breathing seemed to be changing, so I thought it would not be long. However, I was spectacularly wrong. Monty stirred, awoke and requested to go for a cigarette!

Just as the moment of dying is unpredictable, so also it is difficult to know when or indeed whether to leave the dying person's bedside. Sometimes the family, if they are present, will guide you in this, inviting you to stay for the duration, at other times it is best to leave them to themselves. Each situation requires a sensitivity and empathy which I hope, as pastors, we acquire from experience. In Sally's case, it felt right to stay, and the family wished us to. We drank tea, we chatted about Sally and about her life, as well as getting to know her adult children. We talked to Sally too, and the family held her hand or stroked her arm, as she lay. We stayed until the moment of her death, and for a while afterwards. In Monty's case, once I realized that his death was not imminent, it was certainly time to go home and back to bed!

Often when the end is very close, there comes a time when voices become more hushed, and eventually cease altogether. In my experience this can be a moment of tranquillity but also great heartache. We wish the pain, if there is any, to be over for the dying person, and we wish the emotional pain for us as the watchers to be over too. Accompanying these strong emotions can also be guilt—for willing someone to die; for being too selfish; or for not wanting them to go. There is no doubt at all that accompanying the dying person as a friend or relative is one of the most testing and intense emotional experiences most of us will ever encounter.

I have been with several people as they have died who have seemed to need permission to go. I have known people wait for the right person to appear, or for all the family to gather, or conversely to take their last breath when they are left alone for the briefest interval. I recall travelling across London to a hospital where the father of one of the prisoners was dying. The prisoner had been given special leave to be in the hospital, and had asked me to be present. When I arrived at the bedside where all the extended family was gathered, I introduced myself to the family and to the father. I remember his daughter saying, "It's OK Dad, Rosie's here now." I then told him that I was going to say some prayers. I started saying the Lord's Prayer, and before we reached the end, he had died. I was only in the room a few minutes.

I believe that sometimes the dying person has some control over the moment of death, and that for some hearing words from loved ones, saying it is all right for them to go, that the family will be OK, this is enough for them to stop resisting and let go of battling to stay alive. I also believe that no matter how unresponsive someone may seem as they are dying they can hear what is being said around them. I believe that this is really important for families of those gathered around the bedside to be aware of, so that if there are things they wish they could have said before, it is not too late to say them now.

Dying, of course, brings many regrets for the things we have said, or things we have done which we wish we hadn't. If one is fortunate enough to reach the dying person in time, then saying those things, even without the possibility of discussion, feedback or even forgiveness being offered, can ease the burden of sorrow and guilt a little. It may also ease the burden of letting go for the dying person—though that, of course, will never be known or understood.

I also believe that as someone is dying there is a conversation and experience they may be having which is totally beyond our comprehension in this dimension of our existence. My own belief is that there is a compassionate creator engaged in a dialogue with the dying person as they move from one existence into another realm. I also believe, and have seen on more than one occasion, the dying person appear to be extending their arms and appearing to look and see something which I cannot see, as if they are engaged with someone else, or reaching out to them. I know people who have had near death experiences sometimes talk of being drawn to a white light or warmth. What we now surmise and observe from those who are dying, we will, of course, only really know from our own experience.

I was particularly struck by this when visiting an elderly prisoner who was dying. He'd been a stoker on steam ships, had had an incredibly hard existence and was a cantankerous old so-and-so. He was as grumpy in dying as he was in living, but nevertheless I enjoyed my visits to him. One thing a priest should not be afraid of is speaking the truth, and so when someone is close to death, I don't skirt around the issues or pretend that the inevitable isn't happening. I think sometimes people find this reassuring. They know that if I don't mind mentioning the D word, then they can talk about it too—their fears, their regrets, their hopes. Stan was adamant that he didn't care, and didn't believe in anything beyond. I wasn't in the business of trying to convert him, or change his mind; that would have been a gross misuse of my position, and his vulnerability. I did let him talk, and I did tell him my reflections and beliefs; we agreed to differ! Then there came the stage when he moved beyond words. I still visited him then, just to sit and wait with him, and on more than one occasion I watched him extending his arms towards something or someone that I could not see, but he clearly sensed.

Accompanying someone in their final hours is helped when one already has a relationship with them. As prison chaplain one of the roles is to visit the hospital wing every day. This meant that if prisoners were in our hospital wing for any length of time, I often got to know them even if I hadn't encountered them previously on the wings. One of our residents in the hospital wing was Larry. Over the several years he spent in the prison hospital we had plenty of time to converse—about his love of fishing, his taste in music, his family, his interest in trains, and his hopes for the future. As his health deteriorated the conversations changed from his dreams of release to the prospect of dying. It is one of the greatest fears of prisoners when they come into prison that they will die there, and when prisoners arrive in prison in their later years, in their sixties, seventies and sometimes eighties, often for historic offences, there is a strong likelihood that this will happen.

I knew from my conversations with Larry that he was frightened of dying, and of being alone as he died. The prison tried to be as compassionate for prisoners in their final days as is possible within the regulated circumstances of a prison. When someone is very close to the end, the door of their room is left unlocked, so nursing staff can spend as much time with them as they need or the patient desires. I knew Larry's concerns, and I also knew of his love of singing and the hymns he particularly liked to sing. So there were occasions when he was dying and no longer able to converse when I sat with him and sang hymns. It reminded me of singing to my children as they fell asleep when they were infants. Of course, I will never know whether this helped Larry, but I know that by singing familiar tunes quietly we were able to create an atmosphere of calm and tranquillity which I hope eased his anxiety about the process.

In many pastoral circumstances of great sorrow, or distress, the only genuine response to another's pain is silence. There are times when we move beyond words in our compassion, and anything we might try to say sounds hollow and banal. You cannot use platitudes to cheer up someone who is dying. You cannot pretend to someone who is aware that they are approaching death that they are wrong, although I know people who might try this—probably more to make themselves feel better than to empathize with the patient. In my experience it can be more compassionate to listen than to speak, and to wait alongside in companionable silence can be comforting to someone who is dying. In the busyness of life, we are not used to waiting, but when we are dying or with someone who is dying, there is often nothing but waiting to be done. As a pastor it is so important to wait, and to not be in a hurry to leave if someone needs company.

In a prison, those who are dying rarely have the opportunity to spend any length of time with their loved ones; even if families want to visit, and some may not, there are restrictions on the amount of time they can spend. There have been occasions where I have spent several hours, simply sitting with a dying prisoner, knowing their fear of being alone, and knowing that there is no one else coming to spend time with them. Nurses will also do this when they have the time, but they have other duties with prisoner patients. The chaplain has nothing else more pressing to do, and they can give the gift of time.

Pastoral care requires travelling with someone at their pace. One prisoner, Charles, had been in our hospital wing on several occasions. He had had several episodes of cancer in his life and had fought back from them with determination. Whilst in prison his cancer returned and was treated, and each time he faced it with the same resolution to get better. He continued to hold this view that he would recover despite others being clear that his condition was now incurable. If someone like Charles holds these strong views which are at odds with reality, it is a delicate path to tread. On the one hand his views need to be respected and he needs to keep a sense of hope, but on the other hand he needs to recognize the possibility that he will die, and if feasible prepare himself and others for that eventuality. What one can of course say for certain is that everyone will die one day, and that getting ready for it is something everyone must do, whether or not they have been given a diagnosis. Right until the end, Charles found it hard to acknowledge that he was dying or to talk about how he felt, but I always kept the door open to him having this conversation should he wish to do so.

I have met many people who are dying who seem to find it difficult to talk about it with their loved ones, or with staff. I observe that this seems to be more common with men than women, and often they are men who are very practical. What transpires in conversation, though, is that the person who is dying has sorted out all the finances, left lists of passwords, or has completed all the DIY in the house to their satisfaction. This is a way of preparing and recognizing the inevitability of death without the need to talk about it, and their way of making it as easy and comfortable for those they are leaving behind as they can.

In my experience those who believe that there is something of meaning beyond death often face their own mortality with greater acceptance and openness. When someone who has a strong faith is dying, there is more opportunity to talk about their feelings about what may be to come. This doesn't mean that they don't have fears, regrets or sadness about those they are leaving behind; these are natural human feelings which even the person with the strongest faith may encounter.

When another of our parishioners, Chris, was diagnosed with terminal cancer, I had the great privilege of taking Communion to her in her home regularly. Her daughter was always present on these occasions, so it gave me the opportunity to build up a relationship with her as well. People are sometimes surprised that when someone knows they are dying they can remain cheerful and laugh. It was certainly the case with Chris. She was always cheerful in her life, though it hadn't been an easy one, and was going to die in the same frame of mind. Chris taught me that one's approach to life and death can be seamless; whether living or dying, you are the same person throughout. Chris was one of my many tutors in how to be alongside someone at the end of their life. She saw that I was anxious about my own ability to cope with loss and she eased it for me.

When one has known someone for a period of time, especially when it has involved them facing their own death, it can be hard to face the time when you know that you will not see that person again. I have always dreaded goodbyes that are final, and there is nothing that seems more final than saying goodbye at the end of a visit to someone who is close to death. As a pastor there are of course boundaries which must be maintained, but as people we are all vulnerable, and there are times when expressing one's sadness and making oneself vulnerable is the only option. I have cried with a person who is dying, or with their relatives, but I hope I have always maintained awareness that this is their grief and not mine, and that the last thing they need is for me to hijack their experience of sorrow by becoming overwhelmed. This is when having time to reflect and process one's own feelings away from the immediate situation is very important and having wise and caring people to support me has been essential throughout my ministry.

Holy dying

One of the most profoundly important and formative experiences of my early ministry was in accompanying an elderly priest, Father Pat, in the final months and days of his life. The lessons I learned from him have stayed with me and have shown me the value of seeing opportunities for learning in every encounter. I believe this experience has shaped and formed me into the priest I have become. What I have also learned is that even when words are no longer possible, the one who is dying can be our tutor, and can give us great gifts to treasure.

> [w]hen you grow old, you will stretch out your hands, and someone else will fasten a belt around you and take you where you do not wish to go.
>
> *John 21:18*

I often thought of this passage when as a curate I visited Father Pat in a residential home in our parish. I'd only known him in the latter years of his life when verbal communication was getting progressively harder, and his mobility and ability to do things for himself were very restricted.

It didn't take long, however, to realize that I was in the company of a great man of prayer, as well as someone with a lasting sense of humour. I always felt incredibly humbled when visiting Father Pat; here was I, a young, fresh-faced curate, sitting alongside one of such vast pastoral experience and spiritual depth. I think this was the most moving part of my vigil with Pat as he was dying, that just as I was waiting with him, so he must have waited with many of his parishioners when they were facing death.

Father Pat always affirmed me in my ministry. I sensed his support of me as deacon, and then as priest. At the end of each visit I always asked him to give me a blessing, and though I couldn't always make out the words, I knew the intention was strong, and indeed I felt that I had been blessed by God through him. It was a great joy to me to be able to bring Father Pat the sacrament of Holy Communion, and it was particularly special to me that he was present on one occasion when I presided at the Eucharist in our church.

On Ash Wednesday, in 1998, I visited Father Pat at the same time as the chaplain to the home where he was resident. The three of us said prayers together, since Father Pat had been unable to attend the service in the chapel earlier in the day. I decided then that it would be part of my Lenten discipline to visit Father Pat more regularly than I had managed to do previously. I always prefer to take something up, rather than give something up, in Lent. I had no idea then that these would be my final visits, many of them to hospitals, and would mean accompanying him to the point of death.

It says in the ordinal (the priestly instructions you assent to when becoming ordained) that a priest should prepare the dying for their death.

Father Pat and I had sometimes talked about death, and how the waiting for it seems so long drawn out. I knew Father Pat was ready to die, but sometimes God's timing isn't ours. I like to think that we die when we are called, and if death doesn't come soon enough for us it may be because we still have lessons to learn, or people to teach. Perhaps I was one of Pat's students?

In his book *The Stature of Waiting*, W. H. Vanstone talks of the Passion narrative of Jesus in the Gospels as being the move from activity to passivity; being rather than doing. It is an incredibly hard process to undergo, especially for those who have spent their lives being carers or doers. And yet it is an immensely important time for it throws us back onto our reliance on God, since there is little else left that we can do.

In hospital when one is very sick, one can only wait and be dependent. One has no control. When Pat moved from his care home to hospital, he had to be moved by the nurses, so that he didn't get bedsores, and he had drips for nourishment and catheters. In his pyjamas, and removed from his beloved books and pictures, he was just another patient in another bed. And for those of us who waited by his bedside, it did seem unfair and cruel for him to have to be like this for so long. To pray for healing in this situation was to pray for Pat to be relieved of his suffering and to die.

And yet day after day we waited; through Holy Week to Maundy Thursday. On this day it is traditional to have a vigil, mirroring Jesus in the Garden of Gethsemane. It felt entirely appropriate to me to spend my time of vigil not in church but at the bedside of Father Pat. I simply sat with him as he slept. It seemed to me that the body of Christ was as manifest and as holy in the broken body of one of his saints as it was in the sacrament on the altar. And it was as hard to sit with this dying man as it must have been for the disciples to sit and wait with Jesus in the Garden.

After that night I had a feeling that Pat would die on Good Friday, but God, and Pat, had better timing, and knew that Pat would see in Easter Day. It was right that he should, and on Easter Sunday, as I sat with him once again, I must have known that this would be my last visit. Though I wept that he was still with us and in such pain, perhaps I was weeping for this being a final farewell; for though in my head I wished for death as a solution, no ending is without sorrow and the pain of saying goodbye.

On this last visit, an immensely important one for me, I expressed my feelings of helplessness to Pat. Nothing can prepare you or train you to sit with someone as they die. I was there alone, apart from the angels, and I had no sense of whether what I was doing was right, or helpful, or of value. I wanted so much Pat's reassurance, I wanted his wisdom and pastoral expertise, and I felt completely inadequate. I know Pat understood my vulnerability then, he looked at me as I wept, and I glimpsed a tear in his own eye too. In that moment I knew that all I have to bring to being a priest is who I am, and in that instant, I was being fully me, and Pat, and I'm sure God, understood. Father Pat died in the early hours of Easter Tuesday.

The only other priest I have accompanied in his death was my father. I was always very close to my Dad, and as a child one of my greatest fears was losing him. While it may be one thing to accompany parishioners, it is a different thing altogether to be alongside a family member as they die. The personal outweighs the professional, and I felt as vulnerable and fragile as anyone else in this position. However, the one thing I did have which others in my family did not, was the experience of being with someone who is dying and knowing what death can look like. So, when my father was moved from hospital to a hospice, I felt it my role for the family to offer to be with him.

I was terrified and awed by doing this, but I somehow felt compelled and at peace about it too. When my father was first diagnosed with cancer four years earlier, I remember visiting him in hospital. Seeing him on a ward in the hospital all connected to tubes and looking so frail and elderly, I cried and told him that I wasn't ready to lose him yet. We both cried, and he said that he wasn't ready to go yet either. Thanks to the medical care and chemotherapy we then had four years of getting ready for the inevitable, having conversations which we might never have had, and making memories with all the extended family. So, when the end was really near, it felt different.

When I approached Dad in the bed in the hospice, this time I was ready. However, my father knew how hard I had found it before, and his first question when I told him I had come to be with him and to stay was "Are you all right with this?" He didn't need to say with his dying, for we both knew what he meant. Without a moment's hesitation, I said "Yes", and I knew I was. Four years before I had had little experience of people dying, but my role as chaplain at HMP Isle of Wight, where we had high numbers of prisoners' deaths, had given me so much more experience. It was as if all my ministry to date had been to prepare me and enable me to do this one final thing for my father, and for the family.

If you cannot die in the comfort of one's own bed, then a hospice is the best place to die. There the staff know that the most important things are for the patient to be as comfortable as possible and to have as much quality time with those they are leaving as they can. The nurses put up a camp bed for me in Dad's room and let me spend all my time with him. We were able to say prayers together and talk and be silent together. I remember when we came to say the Lord's Prayer, I stumbled over the phrase "Thy will be done", for it seemed so hard for God's will to be to take Dad from me. I squeezed Dad's hand then, and we both were able through tears to carry on.

I had taken some conkers from my parents' garden to the hospice, as a reminder of their home, and in those hours when I was with Dad and it was hard and sad, I held on to them tightly and squeezed them to distract myself from the emotional pain. I shared this idea with my nieces when they came to see Dad for the last time and found it so hard to say goodbye.

I am so glad that I was able to spend that time with my father. It was a richly precious time, which I know many others may not have been so fortunate to share with their loved ones. I know that Dad would have been comfortable dying on his own if none of us had felt able to be with him. He believed so strongly that he was not alone, that God was with him, and he was so generous and kind that he would not have wanted to cause any of his family unnecessary suffering. But in the end, in his final hours both my sisters and mother felt able to join us, and we had a very special few hours with Dad as he seemed in a deep sleep. It felt as if we had gone beyond words, though we talked to him and prayed with him, sang songs and reminisced. Then we sat in silence and waited, watched and waited. Dad's breathing changed, and to my astonishment I realized that with each out breath he was saying a series of four single words, "Thy will be done." He repeated it over and over, until he stopped breathing and died.

I believed at the time that Dad was praying to God as he died. But now I also believe that Dad was giving us a gift, and knowing how I had struggled with this part of the Lord's Prayer earlier, I believe it was a message of hope to me in particular. Those who are dying have so much still to teach and to share if only we can listen closely and learn. I felt so moved and touched by the beauty and wisdom in Dad's death that I felt compelled to preach about it at a memorial service for him a few weeks later. It is also perhaps why I am writing this book.

CHAPTER 4

Disturbing Deaths

In the previous chapter I described what a good death can look like. In this chapter I will look at death in some of its most disturbing forms: death in youth and death that is self-inflicted. I will consider how those affected by suicide experience shame and ask whether the Christian tradition has offered or could offer help. I use the story of Judas Iscariot to explore these issues theologically.

Death comes in many forms. Not every death is neat; not every dying is planned and prepared for. Many will die alone, too soon, violently, unexpectedly or unloved. Thousands will die in conflicts, natural disasters, or as a consequence of poverty, hunger or disease. Each different circumstance of death generates different emotions, responses and grief in those connected to them. I draw here on my own personal experiences of disturbing deaths particularly from my work as a prison chaplain.

Suicide in prison

I vividly recall the first suicide in prison which I was heavily involved in. I had been at a multi-disciplinary meeting on the healthcare wing in Holloway Prison, when a member of the nursing team came in and asked for assistance. She was calm and matter of fact, but there was something about her which showed to all of us in the room that there was something of significance happening at that moment. I remember catching the eye of another person in the room, and together we left to see what was going on.

We hurried down the corridor to the prisoner's room. Already there were nurses present, and one was attempting to revive the woman with mouth-to-mouth resuscitation. I couldn't see much, but I knew the woman on the bed, and the nurses attending to her. There was no panic, but urgency and intensity. I know my limitations, and I know that having too many people around can only confuse and obfuscate what needs to be happening. It is better to stand back and take on the role of runner than to gawp and get in the way. The nurses were asking for a doctor, so I made it my place to try to contact someone.

In the end, there was nothing to be done; the woman had taken her own life, and no other action by those around would have prevented this from happening. At the time, of course, and for months afterwards, there is the constant soul-searching: could I have done more? If I had gone past her room instead of going in the other direction, might I have seen her and talked to her to distract her? Had she shown signs of wanting to do this which I had missed? Did she intend to do it, or was it a tragic cry for help which went horribly wrong?

In a prison setting, every death of a prisoner becomes a crime scene. There is intense scrutiny and analysis of everyone's actions. A prison is a closed community, and therefore there could always be the possibility of an abuse of power or even violence by those who hold the keys, or indeed by another prisoner. So, despite every effort being made to save a prisoner's life, often the staff become acutely conscious of their own part in case they have made a mistake. Every death in custody has a coroner's inquest, and families will have many questions they want answering through this process.

A chaplain who is around at the time of a death in prison can provide a listening ear to staff and others caught up in the situation. As with any death there is often anger from those left behind. Why did they do it? Why didn't they tell me it was getting bad? Why didn't someone stop them? Why didn't they get her help before? Why did she come to prison in the first place when she was clearly so vulnerable? Of course, there cannot be any answers at this stage, and sometimes there never will be, but giving people the time and space to voice these feelings can be an invaluable outlet for their grief.

Many times, I have found myself making endless cups of tea for those who have been involved in this kind of situation. There is shock and disbelief once the adrenalin has passed and the outcome has become clear. Some staff will feel that they need to be professional, especially in front of prisoners, or even their colleagues. Sadly, some staff have encountered so many deaths in their time of service that they feel they are immune. Some almost pride themselves that they are so boundaried or hardened that it doesn't have an impact on them any more. However, this could be one death too many that they have encountered, or it may trigger other experiences and memories which make this situation more difficult to deal with emotionally. By listening attentively, it may be possible to pick up warning signs of emotional fatigue and burn-out.

Some newer staff who experience a suicide for the first time may feel they have to show to their colleagues that they are all right, otherwise they might be considered to be weak. Some have dreaded this experience happening and have wondered how they will cope, so they may feel some kind of relief that at least they have been through it now, rather than fearing it happening. Letting people express whatever they feel without judgement is essential in any pastoral situation, and when facing a traumatic death this is definitely the case.

Fellow prisoners also need time to process and deal with this kind of trauma. When a prisoner makes a serious attempt to take their own life, the rest of the prisoners will be removed from the situation to enable those that need to be dealing with it to be unhindered. This can mean other prisoners are locked in their rooms, while they can hear the sounds of action outside. I can't begin to imagine how this must feel. To hear noises of running or shouts, and to be left only with your imagination about what is going on, can be very disturbing. Those who have been in the rooms next to the prisoner who has taken their own life or died in some other way may even have heard distressing sounds before the staff have appeared. They may or may not have alerted staff. Their feelings may be very complicated, and yet often they may not be told anything until the immediate situation has been resolved, hours later.

Sometimes those of us who are not directly involved in the medical needs of the prisoner can spend time listening to other prisoners, possibly through the door of their locked room, and though we cannot discuss what is happening at the time, we can at least reassure them that everything that can be done is being done and that they will be told as soon as it is possible to do so. So many prisoners experience thoughts of wanting to end their own life, even if they never act on these, that the knowledge that someone else whom they may have known has attempted and been successful in doing so must generate many complex thoughts and feelings.

In hospital when someone dies, there is generally the dignified response of the nurses in laying that person out. It is a way not only of honouring the dead, but is also I believe a healing ritual for those who have cared for them. In a prison when there is a death, this is not possible. No one is allowed to touch the body, and no last rites are administered. I know that nurses in prison are frustrated that they can't carry out their role as they would wish. In prison following any death the police are called, the room is sealed, and only the coroner can enter the room. Occasionally when I have been present at a death scene, after the coroner has been and the body has been formally identified, I have been permitted to stand in the entrance of the doorway and say some prayers, but I have not been allowed to touch the body. I know that sometimes the knowledge that someone like myself has said a prayer with the deceased can help a grieving family member or another prisoner or member of staff.

A death by suicide can often be a scene of great disturbance. Those who are first at that scene may experience shock and revulsion at what they see. Though staff may act very professionally at the time, the aftermath of what they have witnessed can stay with them for days or months afterwards. The feelings that accompany these experiences need careful attention, and I have found many staff in prison who suffer to some degree from post-traumatic stress. Staff may not only relive the events of this particular incident over and over again, but one incident can trigger recollections of previous experiences like this.

I was called to the prison late one evening, when a young prisoner had died. I was there simply to be a presence and offer support where I could. I clearly recall the moment when the funeral director arrived and took the young man's body away. Although I was at some distance from the scene, sitting with a member of staff, I was struck by the sound of the zip on the body bag; my own sense of hearing was heightened at that moment. Having worked in prisons myself for sixteen years, I have the utmost admiration for prison officers, whose job is often not recognized or valued in the same way as other public services.

I remember another death in custody in which I was very involved. It was with a young woman called Amy, with whom I had had some pastoral conversations. Her state of mind had been of sufficient concern to staff for her to be under a greater level of observation, where she was being checked on at regular intervals to ensure that she was safe. But even the best safeguards cannot prevent someone from taking their own life if they are determined to do so. Prisoners time the visits of staff to their door, so that they have the maximum amount of time to take any action. This may have been the case with Amy.

There is no set action for a chaplain in the circumstances of a serious attempt at suicide, and on this occasion, as I happened to be on the wing where the prisoner was, I became very involved. When the paramedics indicated that they would take Amy to the hospital, hoping against hope that they could revive her, I was able to offer to go in the ambulance with her. This was to prove a great support to the family with whom I would engage in the aftermath. It helped them to know that their daughter was not alone in her final moments, and that someone neutral like myself was accompanying her through her final stages of life. Sadly, Amy did not recover and was pronounced dead at the hospital. I was able to stay with her when all the interventions were finished, and I said prayers with her.

Later that day, I accompanied a governor of the prison to meet the family. There is no easy way of breaking bad news to a family in any circumstances, but to have to tell parents that their daughter has taken her own life in prison is incredibly hard. I can visualize that scene in immense detail as I write, though it is now more than thirteen years ago. I suppose any experience of trauma stays with you in intensity and though you move on from it, you can recall it vividly when bringing it to mind again. The process of grief affects people in different ways. Amy's mother was distraught and tearful, whereas her father was enraged. Amy's mother wanted to know that her daughter was not alone and had been cared for; her father wanted someone to blame. Amy's parents continued to react in these different ways for months, and even years afterwards, and in addition to the immense loss they had experienced, they struggled to understand and respond to each other's different positions.

There is a huge amount of paperwork, evidence-finding and report-writing that must be undertaken by prison staff in preparation for an inquest, and it may take months or years to come to court. Everyone who has been involved in the care of the individual is questioned by police and may be required to attend. This was the case with Amy's inquest. It occurred nearly two years after her death. It is a long drawn-out and painful period for the family as they are waiting for answers. Those who are called to give evidence may have moved to new jobs. It can be hard to recall the details of the events and actions from so long ago. A family liaison officer is appointed to support the bereaved family from the moment of death until the inquest and beyond. This is the link person through whom the family can ask questions and make contact with the prison staff. I went to the inquest, partly because I had been involved with Amy shortly before her death and so was required to give evidence; but also because I had been offering support to her family, and to staff who had been affected by her death.

Dying too soon

Any death brings sadness and grief, but when someone dies in older age those who are bereaved can find some comfort that their loved one has lived a long life, and that this is the natural course of events. When a child dies, or when someone dies at a young age, there is additional pain of the loss of the future.

In my own family, my sister's first child, the first grandchild, the first of the next generation, was born with multiple health needs which meant that his life was going to be very short. This event of his birth, so joyously anticipated in the family, became very soon an immensely sorrowful situation. I was 17 at the time of his birth, and I was away from the family when he was born. I received the news of his birth and his frailty within the same phone call. It is hard to describe the mixed feelings of shock and anger at this news. I remember pacing around the room of the place where I was staying, crying and kicking the furniture. This was the first great sorrow I had ever experienced, and the emotional pain created a great physical reaction. I cannot begin to imagine how my sister and her husband coped with this news. Tom's life, six short weeks, was one of great love and compassion. He was able to come home for some of this and received endless cuddles and warmth.

When you look back at a sad experience from the distance of time, it is hard to recapture completely the pain, for as you move through the stages of grief, and life develops in new ways for all who are involved, your perception of what you experienced also alters. But for any who have lost children more recently than this, I am sure the memories and trauma are more real and raw.

In Tom's case we could comfort ourselves that his life was precious, that he never knew anything but love, and that he was not in pain. When parents have to witness and accompany their children through ongoing physical discomfort or illness, this must cause additional suffering and heartache.

A prisoner's son was in a special school, and I went with her when she was allowed to visit him. He had been a normal, boisterous, active small boy, whose life was changed horrendously when he caught fire in his home. His burns were so severe that he was hospitalized, with severe brain damage and immobile for the rest of his life. He was prone to infection, and his life constantly hung by a thread. All parenting carries guilt and self-analysis. Charlie's mother carried many additional burdens. Could she have prevented it happening? What if . . . ? What if . . . ? If only . . . . Such was her pain that she found it difficult even to visit him and to be with him, knowing, as she must have done, what he was like before, and comparing him with how he was now.

While his mother was in prison, the school called to say that Charlie was deteriorating and that they expected him to die soon. I went with her to see him. Charlie's mum came from a very religious family, and so she and her relatives found some comfort in the prayers that we said around his bedside. Perhaps because the family had lived with the possibility of Charlie's death for so long, the reality of it when the time came was something of a relief, though for a family to admit this at the time is practically unthinkable.

When someone dies young or unexpectedly, there is the added distress of not having said what you would have wanted to say or sometimes having said things which you regret. There may be no time to prepare for the death, and there is the additional painful loss of the future. Since most of us have plans and hopes, desires of what we might do when we get older, or even where we might go on holiday next year, suddenly all these aspirations are snatched from us, along with the individual themselves. A young partner can feel cheated of not only the person they have loved, but the future they had anticipated together.

Often those who have not experienced loss don't really know what to say. They may avoid talking about the death, or they may try to hurry the person along in their grief. Some people told my sister that she was young and that she could have other children. This was not helpful in the least and makes me angry even now to think that people, well-meaning though they may be, can be so crass. I have heard many times in my pastoral ministry, of people who have struggled with accepting the death of a loved one being told by others that they should be over it by now. It is as if those who have never experienced a loss are experts on the process of grieving and judge the progress or otherwise of others on this journey. Some people think that grief has a time limit and that after a certain time it should be finished. The reality, as anyone who has lived through the loss of a loved one will know, is very different.

In the hospice some of the hardest deaths for the staff to process are when the patient is young, around the ages of the nurses and doctors who are caring for them, or when they are of a similar age to their children or grandchildren. On the ward sheet, which is printed daily, the age of each patient is always given. I find myself looking at this and thinking that they are my age or younger, and it makes me acutely aware of my own mortality. I am certain that others do the same. But age is not really an indicator of how we will approach our own death. I have met people in their forties who have accepted the fact that they are dying, and people in their nineties who have not. Perhaps death comes too soon for most of us, and most of us have unfinished business, things we have put off, or not had the opportunity to do, even in our advancing years.

Death wish

Most people will identify with death coming too soon. However, for some people, death cannot come soon enough. In prison there are much higher numbers of people with mental health problems than in the general population. Some people with psychosis will hear voices telling them to kill themselves; some with depression or anxiety will not want to exist. Some of these people will struggle with self-harm and many will have suicidal thoughts which they attempt to act upon. Not everyone who self-harms wishes to be dead; some already feel dead and by cutting themselves and seeing blood they are reminded that they are alive. Some need to feel physical pain in order to distract themselves from the emotional turmoil inside. For many, self-harm has become an addiction from which it is hard to escape. Some feel comfort from the nurturing they need to give to themselves or receive from others once they have self-harmed; some crave attention.

As I said earlier, women account for a high proportion of reported self-harm incidents in prison. I have learned a great deal about self-harm from working with women in prison, where the incidents of self-harm are frequent and often extreme. Often self-harm is connected to abuse; invariably it is associated with poor self-esteem, even self-loathing. Often it is accompanied by addiction to drugs or alcohol; these life choices in themselves can be forms of self-harm.

Sarah was a prolific self-harmer. She was serving a life sentence in Holloway Prison, where she had lived for several years before I first met her, in our healthcare unit. Sarah had very little in her life that gave her pleasure. Before coming to prison, she was an alcoholic. She was a football fan and supported Arsenal. She would have been a chain smoker in prison, if funds had allowed. Instead she bought what little tobacco she could and scrounged the rest. She could be seen during the hour's exercise she received daily, wandering around the yard searching for cigarette ends; it was a pitiful sight. Sarah's main object in life seemed to be negotiating how to get her next cigarette or thinking of ways to kill herself. Each time she made a serious attempt on her life or self-harmed by burning herself with a lighter or setting light to her hair, she was placed on constant watch, with a member of staff sitting outside her door all the time. Sarah had very little to live for; she had no one to visit her, no friends making contact with her at all. Her life was barren and bleak, and no amount of cajoling or persuasion helped her to change. She refused all therapeutic input, though she did go to the art room on a few occasions. As chaplains we visited the healthcare wing every day, so I got to know Sarah quite well. Conversation was limited, because Sarah's interest in life, and her sphere of reference, were so small. I do remember her telling me once that the one thing she wanted to do was to walk in the rain. In HMP Holloway, if it was wet, exercise—as an hour in the fresh air was called—was cancelled.

I left Holloway in 2002 to take up a post in another women's prison in Surrey. A few months later I was at a meeting in central London. The chaplain who had replaced me in Holloway was due to be there, but his colleague informed me that he had had to go and take a funeral for a prisoner. As she told me this, I immediately knew that the prisoner who had died was Sarah. I believe she was being moved from one prison to another. She had had a stopover in another prison on the way, and that night she had hung herself. So I made an instant decision to abandon the meeting and to go to Sarah's funeral instead. I contacted my chaplain colleague in the prison, who had not yet left the establishment, and asked if I might come and speak at her funeral. It seemed fitting to do so as I had known her well for longer. I wrote my sermon on the bus making my way across London to the crematorium.

Sarah's whole life had been pretty desperate and desolate, and perhaps one might empathize with someone who would want to end this kind of existence by taking their own life. There are others who appear successful and happy, but who also have suicidal thoughts and intentions. Amanda was articulate, intelligent, attractive and employed. She had a good job and prospects. However, she was determined to end her life. Before coming to prison, it seemed that she and her partner had made a pact to take their own lives together; but like a Shakespearean tragedy, the partner had died, and Amanda had not. Amanda was now faced with the double grief of the loss of her love, and the reality of continuing life without them. She was also in prison facing serious charges.

Like Sarah, Amanda was placed on constant supervision. Despite the total invasion of her privacy, the shock of prison itself and her grief,

Amanda maintained a dignified aloofness to her situation. It was as if she knew that whatever external deprivation she experienced, it was as nothing to the inner agony at separation, which she was adamant she would rectify as soon as she could. She chose to end her life slowly and painfully by refusing all food. If there is one thing to increase anxiety in others, it is when someone stops eating. Perhaps our natural instincts tell us to get others to eat. But it was the only thing left to Amanda to control.

I met Amanda on my rounds of the hospital wing. My colleagues had told me about her situation, but I had no idea what to expect on meeting her. I found her very poised and composed, looking fit and healthy. Our conversation might have sounded surreal to many, as we discovered a shared enjoyment of the TV series *The Vicar of Dibley*, and we were able to laugh as we recalled our favourite episodes. Perhaps it was a conversation which normalized an otherwise extraordinary situation, which reminded Amanda, and myself, of her humanity. I also discovered that she had a faith, that she had been brought up in the Anglican Church, and that this had given her life some meaning. After this I would take Communion to her every Sunday after the chapel service, and as we said the Lord's Prayer together, she would receive the host. This was the only thing that would enter her mouth for many weeks.

I have no idea what led to a change of heart for Amanda, but one day she was offered a sweet by another prisoner, and she ate it. From then on, she began to eat normally. She was sentenced and moved to another prison. I had no further contact with her.

A few years later I was attending a conference for chaplains working in the women's estate. I was talking to a colleague who was soon due to retire. Amanda's name was mentioned, and I learned that she had received psychological help, completed her sentence and had been released into new work and accommodation in a new area. However, a few months later she had killed herself. My colleague had taken her funeral.

Although the names and details of the people I write about have been changed to protect their identity, as I write about them and their shocking deaths, each person or their family is clear in my mind, and the tragedy of their situation stays with me still. My involvement with them may have been small, my knowledge of them limited to their experiences in prison, but the sorrow and sadness of their stories remains with me even after many years. How much greater must be the pain for those who knew them well? For all those who have died in similarly distressing circumstances, the grief of those left behind is immense.

Dealing with shame

Those who die by suicide must have been in great distress before taking their own lives, but once the act has happened it is others who will feel this pain so acutely. The families and friends of someone who has taken their own life will be left with confusion and innumerable questions. Anger is part of the processing of any grief, but the anger which may be felt when a loved one kills themselves makes grieving very complicated. Families often feel vast amounts of anger at the deceased, and then they may feel guilty for doing so. On the one hand they want to rage at the person who has died, and yet they feel their own pain acutely and feel further enraged with their loved one for inflicting this on them. They may be aware of the pain their loved one went through in order to reach this decision but they may be angry that they didn't come to them for help, or angry with themselves for not seeing this coming. They may feel that the suicide was a selfish act, which took no account of how those left behind would feel. They may feel guilty for feeling angry, but at the same time feel overwhelmed with sadness and sorrow, for their loved one and for themselves.

They may also feel tainted by the experience of loss in this way and imagine that others will hold them responsible for their relative's actions, as if they have somehow driven them to it. They may not get the same kind of sympathy from others; indeed they may feel ostracized and excluded from society as their grief and situation is so shocking. Families may experience years of anger, pain and darkness as they struggle to come to terms with what has happened.

In the process of writing this book I met a woman who had experienced two suicides in her family forty-five and thirty years ago. The trauma of these events was still as vivid as if it was much more recent, and she, like so many, needed to narrate the story of these family tragedies. What was so apparent was that the distance of time had done little to alleviate her feelings of guilt and responsibility. The "what ifs" and "if onlys" were still as strong now as they were when the deaths first occurred. In addition to the pain of the losses she had experienced there was also the distress caused by the reactions of those around her. As a woman of faith herself, she was horrified that her church community and her own minister refused to take the funeral, despite the family member having been active in the church all her life. While this woman was able to hold on to her belief, others in the family never darkened the doors of a church again and turned to other belief systems for solace and support. This woman felt that there had been little change in attitude towards suicides in the fifteen years between these two tragedies. What was also clear from her story was that people in the family reacted in very different ways to these deaths; some never talked of it and kept it a secret from the next generation, while others wanted to be more open and discuss it.

One would hope that there is greater understanding and compassion for people like this woman now than was the case then. I suspect that even with support groups and networks it is still a very lonely and isolating experience losing someone to suicide, because of the trauma of the loss, the violence of the death, the unanswered questions, the self-recriminations, and the social taboos that still surround it.

There is a still a stigma to suicide; the person who has died in this way becomes labelled by their final action, "the son who committed suicide". It is this final act which seems to define them in the eyes of others, as if everything that came before it is eradicated. One mother, when talking of her son, frequently described him in this way to me; it was clearly a habitual pattern when she used his name. How differently would people have reacted or felt if she had said he was killed in a car accident? Despite several conversations with this woman, I felt I never got to know about her son, what he did in his life, what kind of young man he was; only that he had died by killing himself.

The Christian tradition has not helped those who have been bereaved in this way. How appalling that a grieving relative is unable to visit them in the same graveyard where others who have died in a more "respectable" way are buried. How shocking that even today some Christians would tell families bereaved by suicide that their relative has gone to hell. Whatever theological standpoint one may have about the taking of one's own life, it will be those who have loved the person who bear the pain and the shame of it. How appalling that they are made to feel guilty for loving "an outcast". Even though modern attitudes are changing, centuries of legitimized shame linger in the cultural, social and even religious psyche.

In every culture and generation there have been those who have been pushed to the edge of society by the attitudes of others; often they are "put away", so that most people in society do not have to see or think about them; "out of sight and out of mind". In Jesus' time widows, lepers, people with disabilities, mentally disturbed people, were treated in this way. In the Gospels, Jesus is frequently found amongst these people, offering love, healing, forgiveness and new life to them. Jesus challenges the cultural and religious prejudices of his day. Jesus speaks with and heals a disturbed man living amongst the tombs, chained up; he heals a woman who had been ritually unclean for years because of her haemorrhaging; he cures the daughter of a Gentile, because she showed such faith in him; he sees the desperation of a widow whose son has died and brings him back to life.

All these people carried the shame of their society's attitudes. Jesus, in treating them as human beings of worth, not only heals the individuals, he offers healing to society by demonstrating a different way of living which challenges the concept of stigma and shame. How tragic that the gospel message has been so distorted that the Church has for centuries perpetuated exclusion and shaming, not only of those who have taken their own life, but also of their relatives, instead of following the example of Jesus himself and reaching out to them with compassion and love.

Those who die by suicide, and the families who are left behind grieving, remind society of the shadow side of the human condition, the darker part of our existence which we largely try to avoid. To be whole as individuals and as a society we need to identify, embrace and understand the parts of our existence which make us feel uncomfortable, like mental distress and suicide. If we are able to do this we will respond with greater compassion, empathy and emotional maturity to people affected by it.

In 1987 Laurence Whistler, a glass artist, produced an engraved window which he donated to a church in Moreton in Dorset. It depicts Judas Iscariot hanging. The graphic nature of the window meant that the local church and community would not accept its installation, and it became a cause of debate and discussion in the Church and community.

Was it an appropriate image to have in a church? What shocked people more? Was it the depiction of Judas, the one who betrayed Jesus, or was it the depiction of the hanging? Perhaps it was a combination of both. We may have become immune to the images of the crucifixion, or we have sanitized the images of it in our minds, for the cross also depicts a horrific way of dying. If we were to replace the crucifixion with Jesus before a firing squad, or in the electric chair, or in a gas chamber, perhaps we would be reminded of the horror once again?

In 2014, nearly 30 years after its creation, the window was finally installed. It reflected a change in the attitude of the local community towards suicide. Although the window was installed in the church, it cannot be seen from the inside, because the view is blocked by a memorial tablet. The artist's intention was to confine this window to the exterior, making it a shadowy image which can only just be made out, depending on the angle of the light. Perhaps this window is a metaphor for the Church's and society's slowly changing approach to suicide?

The Whistler window has now become something of a place of pilgrimage for those who have been affected by a suicide in the family. It is called the forgiveness window, and as the coins drop from the hand of Judas, some seem to turn into flowers, demonstrating that all is not lost and that there is still hope and the possibility of redemption. Perhaps one day, when people are able to understand suicide and embrace life in the fullness of its complexity, pain, anguish and grief, windows like this will have a place within churches, where the light will be allowed to shine through them completely.

A theological reflection on suicide

Before the Suicide Act in 1961, it was a criminal offence to commit suicide; the families of those who succeeded in taking their own lives could be prosecuted; and those who attempted to kill themselves and failed could be imprisoned. Suicide was considered self-murder.

In the early Christian tradition suicide was considered the ultimate, mortal sin, breaking the sixth of the Ten Commandments, "You shall not kill" (Exodus 20:13, RSV). According to Augustine of Hippo in the fifth century and Thomas Aquinas in the twelfth, it was a denial of God's gift of life and therefore an act of blasphemy. The act of taking one's own life meant that there was no possibility of repentance from the sin, and therefore the perpetrator was left to eternal condemnation. In the sixth century it became law that those who had died by suicide were not permitted to receive a Christian burial on consecrated land. It was only in 2017 that the Church of England finally ended the ban on a full Christian burial for someone who had died by suicide.

Whether or not there has been a softening of doctrine as there is a greater sense of compassion for suicide victims and those affected by it, centuries of negativity towards those who take their own life cannot be easily or swiftly erased. The legacy of shame and guilt that families often feel about their loved ones who have died in this way is enormous. If death itself is still a subject of taboo and avoidance, how much more taboo is death by suicide.

I am sure there are many Christians, like myself, who would want not only to distance themselves from this condemnatory part of the Christian tradition but to divorce themselves from it entirely. As one who has engaged with many people who have felt suicidal, as well as many who have been affected by the death of someone who has taken their own life, I can only feel compassion and sympathy for them. My approach will always be one of pastoral concern and of holding on to the central tenet of my faith that God is Love itself, and as the Psalmist writes:

> The Lord is gracious and merciful, slow to anger and abounding in steadfast love.
>
> *Psalm 145:8*

It is also my belief that there is no place of despair or darkness—emotional, psychological or spiritual—that is beyond the limits of the compassionate God.

> Where can I go from your spirit?
> Or where can I flee from your presence?
> If I ascend to heaven, you are there;
> if I make my bed in Sheol, you are there.
>
> *Psalm 139:7–8*

The most notorious suicide in the Christian story is that of Judas Iscariot, the disciple of Jesus. Judas, who is always labelled in the Gospels as "the one who betrayed" Jesus (Matthew 10:4). I have always felt that the over-emphasis on Judas as the instigator of Jesus' death was unjust, because it was not the action of a single person that led to the crucifixion of Jesus; it was a combination of people, as individuals and groups; including some of the leaders of the Jewish faith and heads of the Roman occupying forces; and the masses of his fickle followers. Neither was Judas the only disciple who let Jesus down; Peter denied him, the others ran away; weren't these actions similarly abhorrent and worthy of condemnation? Perhaps it is more the fact that Judas took money from the authorities to give Jesus away; that he planned the action of betrayal and revealed Jesus to the arresting authorities by a kiss, normally an action of love, which is so shocking. This was a planned act of intention rather than a sign of weakness, fear and human frailty.

Judas has always been remembered for the part he played in Jesus' death. It strikes me, however, that he was still one of the disciples, one of the closest of Jesus' friends and followers, and even if that makes his later actions so abhorrent, Jesus himself must have invited and called him in the first instance to "come and follow me". Did Jesus make a mistake in choosing Judas? Some might argue that Judas was chosen because Jesus knew he was going to be the one who would betray him; I don't hold with this view of a pre-planned, pre-ordained set of events. The action of Judas Iscariot remains associated with his name, because there was nothing he did later to redeem himself. Peter might have been termed "the one who denied Jesus" had he not had the opportunity to be forgiven by the risen Christ and become one of the leading missionaries.

The two significant events that are associated with Judas are that he betrayed Jesus, and that then he was filled with remorse, and he hung himself. What does Jesus himself say to Judas in the Gospel narrative? Indirectly Jesus appears to refer to Judas here at the last supper when he says:

> [w]oe to that one by whom the Son of Man is betrayed! It would have been better for that one not to have been born.
>
> *Mark 14:21*

Some interpretations of this text imply that Judas will face eternal condemnation because of his heinous act, punishment so drastic that it would have been better if he had never been born. But supposing there is an alternative way of reading this text? Suppose Jesus knew the torment and remorse that would accompany the aftermath of the act of betrayal and which would lead the perpetrator to be so full of anguish that he would kill himself? Read in this way, Jesus' statement speaks more of his compassion for the man who would betray him, not of his condemnation of him for the betrayal. This way of looking at the text is much more in keeping with Jesus' approach to others, and it speaks right to the heart of those who are filled with suicidal thoughts and intentions.

Judas, when he saw that Jesus had been condemned, recognized his sin and confessed it to the chief priests. They had no interest in his change of heart or his sorrow; to them Judas had delivered what they had wanted, and he was of no further use to them. The money that he returned to them was a greater dilemma for them than Judas himself. How different it would have been if Judas had been able to acknowledge his sin and shame to Jesus himself? Surely there would have been forgiveness even for Judas, if only the opportunity had been there for him, if only he had been able to live with what he had done?

Peter's denial of Jesus three times is as shocking as Judas' betrayal. We are told in the narrative that Peter, realizing what he had done, wept. If Peter had been of a different personality and temperament, he might have also felt so horrified by his behaviour and his own betrayal of Jesus that he took the same action as Judas. Peter lives with his guilt and shame, however, and no doubt mentally replays his actions again and again in the course of the events of the Passion. Ultimately, Peter is able to be transformed, forgiven and restored by the risen Christ, in a way that Judas could never experience.

By placing Judas and Peter alongside one another in the part they played in the Passion of Jesus, I am highlighting the differences in outlook and perspectives that make up the rich variety of human beings. From my experience of working with people in prison there are some who are filled with remorse for the crimes they have committed; they may be so overwhelmed when faced with the reality and shame of their actions, that they turn their faces to the wall, and long for death, or actively seek it. There are others, however, who when faced with the same level of remorse, seek to live their lives differently, to somehow make amends and in doing so find redemption and restoration. The amount of pain, or self-criticism, or regret any of us can tolerate varies from person to person depending on their make-up, personality and outlook on life.

Jesus approaches people with love and forgiveness; surely, this same attitude and approach would be there for those who are so filled with sadness, despair, emotional and spiritual pain, that they can see nothing of value in remaining alive? Certainly, this is exactly the kind of situation that Jesus' love would seek to connect with. I can imagine Jesus standing alongside someone who is about to jump off a bridge saying: "You are not alone, you are a person of worth, your life has meaning and value, and I love you"; not "This is a terrible mortal sin you are about to commit, and the pain you now feel will be there for eternity because of it!" The tragedy of Judas, and of every suicide, is that they couldn't see, hear, or feel God's love anywhere at that moment. If hell is considered to be separation from God, they were in hell already in the days and hours and minutes leading up to their suicide; they would not be consigned to hell as a consequence after it. Jesus, having full insight into the pain of not feeling loved, and of being so full of regret and shame that you cannot see beyond it, said of Judas:

> It would have been better for that one not to have been born.
>
> *Mark 14.21*

Jesus would have wanted to protect him and spare him the emotional and spiritual torment he would feel afterwards.

I cannot believe that Jesus loved Judas any less than the other disciples who accompanied him in his ministry. He would have been as much part of the family of disciples as any of them. Jesus would have seen and understood Judas as clearly as he saw and understood each of them. He was as aware of Judas' human frailties as he was of the frailties of all his followers. What has always struck me is that Judas was present at the Last Supper, he broke the bread with Jesus, and Jesus washed his feet. Perhaps it was because he was included and shown as much love as the others that the guilt he felt after betraying Jesus was all the more acute. How much easier it is to justify our actions when we feel we have been ostracized, victimized or condemned, rather than when we have felt loved, included and affirmed? How much easier it might have been if Jesus had condemned him as his enemy, instead of calling him "Friend", when he betrayed him with a kiss (Matthew 26:50).

The tragedy of Judas is that he could not bear to remain in the community of followers after his actions; had he done so, then he could also have been a witness to the resurrection. Does that mean that Judas is beyond redemption for eternity? If we return to the Christian tradition, there are some surprises worth reflecting on. In the Apostles' Creed of about AD 390 it states that Jesus was crucified, died and was buried and that "He descended into hell; and on the third day rose again".

This is an astonishing statement. It became known as the Harrowing of Hell, which took place on Holy Saturday, between Good Friday and Easter Day, when Jesus entered hell to set free the righteous who had died since the time of Adam. It was taught in the Early Church and depicted in iconography of the medieval period: for example, *The Harrowing of Hell*, depicted in a fourteenth-century manuscript commissioned by John, Duke of Berry. One icon, *The Resurrection and the Harrowing of Hell* by an unknown Russian artist from the fifteenth century shows a shocking image of Jesus in hell extending his hand of compassion and love to those who inhabited this state. If there is the possibility in early Christian thought that Jesus could enter the underworld of the dead, might there not also be the possibility that Jesus could reach out to Judas from beyond the grave? Surely this is a message of God's love reaching into every part of human experience in this life and beyond. This takes me back to Psalm 139 which I referred to earlier:

> Where can I go from your spirit? . . .
> if I make my bed in Sheol, you are there.
>
> *Psalm 139:7a, 8*

These icons depict a theological truth, that Jesus enters into the darkness of isolation, separation, despair and anguish, not to remain within it, but to shine the light of hope and redemption into it, and to rescue humanity from it.

> The light shines in the darkness, and the darkness did not overcome it.
>
> *John 1:5*

I see the Christian story, and the person of Jesus Christ himself, offering not condemnation to those who died by suicide but offering light and love to those who take their own life or contemplate doing so. If they cannot receive this love in this earthly life, because of the darkness that they feel surrounding them, they can be reached in whatever lies beyond it; for love knows no bounds or limitations, and God is ever-loving. As the apostle Paul writes so beautifully here:

> For I am convinced that neither death, nor life, nor angels, nor rulers, nor things present, nor things to come, nor powers, nor height, nor depth, nor anything else in all creation, will be able to separate us from the love of God in Christ Jesus our Lord.
>
> *Romans 8:38–39*

Conclusions

In this chapter I have reflected on difficult deaths, and particularly on suicide. It is a taboo subject which many feel uncomfortable thinking about but which we all must address as any of us could be affected by suicide at any time. I will refer to taboos at more length in Chapter 9. Those who care pastorally for people must consider what is their theological as well as their pastoral position when faced with someone who wants to end their own life, or has attempted to do so, or when required to support those who have been affected by a suicide in the family.

I had never encountered people who were actively suicidal until I entered prison ministry; I had to develop my own framework for thinking in the distressing circumstances of the moment. By standing alongside those who have been suicidal, or those who have been affected by it, I have witnessed the absolute depths of human misery and sorrow. I have seen people who have no self-worth and no hope that they or their situation can be any different. They have been in a living hell. I have not been able to make it better, or to change the way that they have been thinking, or to rescue them from the depths, and that is a painful reality that anyone who has been affected by suicide has to manage.

I feel immense compassion for the people I have met who have taken their own lives. I feel empathy for them because of the actions they have taken and the distressing thinking which must have led them to do so. I believe God's compassion and love for them is immeasurably greater than we can imagine and that God has known of the struggles and sorrows of each individual completely.

> O Lord, you have searched me and known me.
> You know when I sit down and when I rise up;
> you discern my thoughts from far away.
>
> *Psalm 139:1–2*

Like Jesus reaching out to the dead in the Harrowing of Hell, I believe God's love reaches out to those who are feeling suicidal; the tragedy is that, like Judas Iscariot, they could not grasp it because of the emotional and spiritual pains that overwhelmed them. But "love is stronger than death", and the mercy of God is far greater than humanity can ever comprehend.

In the painting by Sieger Köder described in Chapter 1, there is a young woman sitting on the edge of the steep well; perhaps she is contemplating taking her own life by throwing herself in? The well is very dark and deep, and could symbolize the depths of despair which those who have contemplated suicide, or who have been affected by it, feel. The woman is looking into the darkness alone, and that is no doubt how she and those who feel the urge to take their own lives feel—totally on their own. Jesus himself experienced this same utter desolation and loneliness on the cross, and cried, "My God, my God, why have you abandoned me?" But as she stares into the water it is not just her own reflection that she sees—there is another reflected face, the face of Christ, gazing up at her. This suggests to me that there is no despairing darkness which we may experience that is not known or understood by God, or in which God's presence may not be revealed.

If I say, "Surely the darkness shall cover me,
and the light around me become night",
even the darkness is not dark to you;
the night is as bright as the day,
for darkness is as light to you.

Psalm 139:11–12

CHAPTER 5

"Good Enough" Deaths

Using case studies from prisons and hospice I ask what does a good enough death mean? Can you die well in prison? Are all deaths in a hospice good? I reflect on pastoral encounters with dying prisoners and with people in a hospice. I use the Passion narrative and Holy Saturday to find a middle way to think about death.

Donald Winnicott (1896–1971), a British paediatrician and psychoanalyst, coined the phrase "good enough mothering" to describe parenting which gives a child all the tools for emotional and psychological development. Having described a good death in Chapter 3 and disturbing deaths in Chapter 4, I am now adapting Winnicott's phrase to refer to dying. I shall consider the relevance of this term in the context of dying in a prison and a hospice.

Should you die well in prison?

It is now enshrined in law that prisoners should have the same access to healthcare, including end-of-life care, as the rest of the community. Having worked in a hospice where the utmost care and attention is paid to the patient who is dying and to their family, I have reflected about the contrasting experience of dying in prison. Is it possible to have a good death in prison? Certainly, one that is self-inflicted is always traumatic and there is no possibility of offering any dignity to the deceased at that moment. But even when death is expected or obviously from natural causes is it possible to show the same respect to the dying and deceased prisoner that would be shown in hospital or at home?

Some argue that a prisoner who has committed a crime forfeits the right to have a dignified death. This assumes prison is for punishment and not reformation and implies that dying well is a privilege for those who have also lived a good and crime-free life. But death is a great leveller; "good people" die tragically, messily and unexpectedly, and "bad people" can have good and peaceful deaths—whether or not they are in prison.

Whatever someone's life experiences, they should be able to receive the same care at the end of life as any other person. If we don't take that approach, then we would be establishing a service for the deserving whilst the rest are left to fend for themselves. We might have criteria for admission into a hospice—where people receive gold-star end-of-life treatment—based on the quality of someone's life rather than their health needs at the time. This would be unethical and at odds with the hospice ethos. To administer a value-based system in end-of-life care would be absolutely impossible and ludicrous.

There are moral, practical and legal imperatives to ensure that prisoners receive appropriate care at the end of life. Fyodor Dostoevsky, in *The House of the Dead* stated, "The degree of civilization in a society can be judged by entering its prisons." Perhaps the care of the dying and deceased prisoner also shows us how civilized a society we are.

Having a good death matters not only for the dying patient but for their family and friends. As Cicely Saunders said, "How people die remains in the memory of those who live on." This is another argument to provide good care to prisoners at the end of life. Even if the prisoner has committed serious offences, their family have not done so, and to them they are still father, mother, child or sibling. The grief for the family of a prisoner may be even more complicated than that of someone in the wider community. It will matter to them that their relative will have received comparable care to the rest of society. The family may be struggling to understand how their relative died when they were in the care of an institution which was supposed to look after them. They may feel additionally let down by the system which failed to protect their loved one adequately. They may suspect that their relative was not able to receive the appropriate healthcare because they were in prison and may suspect that if they had been in the community they might have still been alive. It is because of these kinds of concern that every death in prison is subject to a coroner's inquest.

Can you die well in prison?

I spent eleven years as a chaplain to women in prison. Deaths, which were fortunately few, were tragically always self-inflicted. It was a totally different situation when I arrived at HMP Albany; here I had to exercise a ministry in caring for the dying. While I was there, it had the dubious honour of being the prison where there were the most deaths of prisoners in any prison in England and Scotland; the majority of these were from natural causes. On average we had a death a month.

There are sixteen beds in the purpose-built hospital unit at HMP Albany. Originally this served as an inpatient unit for three separate prison sites in Camp Hill, Albany and Parkhurst. During my time there, Camp Hill closed, and only the Albany and Parkhurst sites were left, which now make up HMP Isle of Wight. There we accommodated about 1,200 prisoners, nearly all of whom were in prison for sexual offences. The hospital wing caters and cares for prisoners with mental health needs, prisoners detoxing and prisoners with chronic or acute conditions. There are also two rooms designated for the use of prisoners at the end of their life.

The employed chaplains were either from different Christian denominations, or Muslim, and one of us, as a statutory duty, would visit the hospital wing every day. We also had part-time and volunteer chaplains in our team, representing most of the main world faiths; they could be called on when necessary to offer pastoral and religious support to prisoners of their faith.

In some ways caring pastorally for prisoners who are dying is the same as caring for anyone at that stage of their lives. But in other ways it is a unique and challenging environment. In Chapter 3, I describe what "a good death" looks like—family around the bedside; pain-free patients; issues resolved; goodbyes facilitated. Is it possible to recreate this in a prison? In a hospital or more especially a hospice, family members can access their loved ones day or night. In a prison, visits take place in a visits hall for two hours when booked, or if possible they can be facilitated on the hospital wing if the prisoner is close to death. Families of prisoners will need to be accompanied at all times and escorted through the hostile confines of a prison environment.

A good death of a prisoner assumes that there are families interested and willing to visit. In HMP Isle of Wight all convicted prisoners serve more than four years, and some have been in custody for decades. Not everyone will have family members still living. Some prisoners may not have been in prison for long, but they have arrived there in their latter years, convicted of historical offences dating back decades. Some prisoners are estranged from their families because of the offences they have committed. Family members may have been victims themselves; families may be divided—those who believe the prisoner to be wrongfully convicted, and others who believe he is rightfully located. Other prisoners may have family, but they may also be in prison elsewhere. Can someone have a good death with all this baggage around?

Every prisoner will face their mortality differently depending on their age, circumstance, previous thinking and approach to life. Just as in hospice not every death is a "good death", so not every death in prison is a "bad death". There may be some prisoners who have a greater social network, more friends and receive better care than they would have done if they had been in the community where their death may have been very lonely, or gone unnoticed or unacknowledged.

Pastoral encounters in prison

I turn my attention now to specific prisoners whom I have supported at the end of life, whose dying and deaths I would describe as "good enough".

Sam was in an outside hospital when I first met him. He had been there for a few days under investigation for his condition. I realized after an hour's visit that here was someone who liked and needed to talk. His biggest fear was that he would be told he had cancer. Shortly after this visit his fears were realized.

It's not easy for anyone when a prisoner is in hospital outside of the prison; the hospital staff, the other patients and their visitors, as well as the prisoner and prison staff. The prisoner is accompanied at all times by two officers, and they are handcuffed to one of them. Even when a prisoner uses the toilet, they are kept on a long chain, so the prison officer is just outside the door. There is no privacy whatsoever. The only time these conditions are relaxed is if the prisoner is immobile and therefore incapable of escaping. It also means that every procedure, every consultation, is overseen and heard by members of prison staff. I am sure this can be as difficult for the prison officers as for the patient. It also means that every reaction to news, good or bad, is observed and monitored. I was alerted to the news Sam had been given and I went back to see him.

Sam described feeling numb when he was told he had cancer, and had great difficulty in taking it in. The consultant told him straight out, without mincing his words, and for that he was grateful. Sam asked if he could have a second opinion, and the consultant replied, "I've told you twice!" By the time I saw Sam a few hours later he had already accepted that to know what was happening was better than the uncertainty and waiting to know; at least he had some idea of what he was dealing with. Such is the power of the human spirit to deal with and assimilate bad news and rationalize and manage it.

On returning to see Sam in hospital that day, neither of us knew of the journey ahead, where it would lead and how it would develop. I simply offered to listen, to attend and to accompany if that was what he wished. Sam was 35. He had been in prison for 20 years. He told me that he came to believe, after about ten years in prison, that he would never be released, but he still had that hope within him that he might. His early life was characterized by violence, physical abuse and emotional neglect. He was, in his own words, out of control. The catastrophic result of this situation was that he murdered a close family member. Twenty years on, after years in secure children's homes, prison institutions and secure mental hospitals, Sam had grown up. Sometimes old patterns of thinking would emerge again, but now he recognized them and fought to shrug them off.

The second time I saw him after his diagnosis, Sam was still in St Mary's Hospital. He was fed up; angry at his situation and angry at being in outside hospital where he felt patronized and feared by some of the nurses. He was desperate to come "home" to prison, where he had his familiar things around him, friends he could reconnect with, and where he could smoke more easily. He was tempted then to fight back, emotionally, to be the horrible, angry individual he used to be; after all he was dying, what was the point in being nice any more? He would still die at the end of it. Feeling angry is a response to loss. But whereas for most of us this would be understood and allowed for, for Sam, to act on these feelings would have been dangerous. I told him he had a choice; how he wanted to die. He couldn't change the fact that he was dying, but he could die well and be respected and affirmed in that, or he could revert to old ways, and die bitter and lonely too.

Sam made that choice. He died well, with great courage and dignity, and most of the time good humour. But he struggled to stay on this track. It is so easy to slip into old habits, to feel sorry for oneself, to think the world owes one a favour, to wish to "curse God and die". But as Sam said, if he did that, then what has the struggle of the last 20 years for? What would all the therapy, the reflection, the offending behaviour courses have really done for him? Did he not owe it to himself, and to those who had helped him on the way, to face this latest challenge as the new Sam rather than the old?

Little did any of us expect that the greatest test of Sam's new outlook on life would come not from the fact of his dying, though that of course brought many challenges, but from facing his victims. Sam had had no contact with his family since his court appearance where he had been sentenced to life in prison. As far as he was concerned his family hated him and wished him dead. However, when he was told that he was dying, Sam was given the option to inform his family of his circumstances; he chose this option, and one of our Family Liaison Officers appointed to his case made contact with them through the Probation Service. Sam and I had many long and involved conversations about his family and his feelings towards them. He was reflective, empathetic and mature about them and himself, but he had no notion of how they had been in the intervening years. It was a momentous occasion when, after an exchange of letters between them, they had their first phone call, and even more so when they asked to come and visit.

Sam and I prepared for this visit by talking. It was clear to me that Sam was still very fearful of his father, a big man who had been a drinker and violent in his parenting. Would his parents and siblings who were visiting wish to kill him for what he had done? When I met Sam's parents in the visits hall just prior to their visit, Sam's parents were equally fearful. Would he still be the angry uncontrollable teenager they had left in care? Did he still harbour murderous thoughts towards them? It was as if each side had an image of the other which had been frozen in time, and neither had any concept or hope that people could change in the intervening twenty years.

Because of my pastoral relationship with Sam, he asked me to stay for this visit with his family, partly for protection, and also because he needed to reflect on this experience afterwards. I have to say that it was one of the most moving and memorable experiences of my ministry, and it brought some measure of healing and reconciliation to most of the family members who participated. Sam saw his Dad as an infirm, vulnerable and softer individual; his parents saw Sam as a mature, reflective and humbled young man. Sam's mum said to him that he would always be her little boy.

The sadness of this situation was that there was not more time available to build on the reconciliation of this visit. But perhaps it is not just quantity of time that matters, but the quality of it. Though there were subsequent letters and phone calls, and though the family hoped to visit again after Christmas, we had to invite them to visit before this as Sam's condition deteriorated rapidly. By the time the visit was arranged, Sam had already slipped into an unresponsive sleep. Though he managed once to open his eyes and acknowledge his parents' presence, Sam could no longer communicate with them, though of course they could with him. I encouraged Sam's mum to give permission for Sam to go, as I felt from my previous experiences of him that this would ease his dying. It was an agonizing moment for Sam's mum, to let go of her child, but she did so with such courage and graciousness, saying that the family member who had died at Sam's hands would be waiting to receive him. This was such a moment of forgiveness and absolution, which no one other than Sam's mother could have offered. Sam did not regain consciousness and died shortly after this visit.

Sam's death was probably as good as it could be in the circumstances. He resolved and addressed many issues which could only have been addressed by the fact of his dying. He ended well with his family, something none of us had anticipated. He was able to view his dying as an adventure—he used this language himself. He reflected on this process and managed his own sense of loss at what might have been. Sam wrote a bucket list while he was dying—things he would have liked to do in his life; they included crossing on a zebra crossing; getting money out of a cash point; having his own place; driving a car and having sex. He was also deeply grateful to the nursing staff in our hospital wing who showed great compassion and tenderness in his treatment, despite the horrific nature of his cancer. I encouraged him to write his thoughts to them and wrote the letter as he dictated it. He included everyone in that letter and had a comment for each of them. He told me once that he played a game in prison, imaging the sort of job a member of staff would do if they were not working in prison. He showed not only an astute ability to observe other individuals, but a great sense of humour! Of all the deaths that happened in our hospital wing, Sam's was probably the most memorable and moving. I told Sam once that I would write about his dying one day. He was pleased to think that he was doing something good with his life, and his death.

There was to be no such reconciliation between Brian and any of his victims. He was a high-profile case, with multiple victims, and few outside prison would regret his passing. Brian had fought the authorities throughout his time in prison, using the vast wealth he had accumulated before coming to prison on solicitors and barristers to fight his case. His main preoccupation on first being told about his prognosis was to guard against those who would get his fortune after he died. Rich or poor, we can't take our possessions with us when we die. For Brian, this was part of the battle he would need to address before he died.

One of the advantages of being a prison chaplain is that people know me, even if I don't know them. They have seen me on the wings, talking to people, leading services or engaging with staff. I may never have spoken to someone until they are in the hospital wing, but they have probably formed an opinion of me before I arrive at their door! For better or worse! Knowing the little I did about Brian, and the conversations staff had about him, I had to work hard on myself to engage with him humanely and genuinely when I first met him in the inpatient unit.

Sometimes "little and often" in pastoral encounters builds up trust quickly. I found that eventually we moved in our conversations from the superficial to the more profound and spiritual. Brain told me that he wasn't afraid of dying; he'd got used to the idea, but he did question what his life, and life in general had been all about. Brian decided to tell me about his childhood, which was spent in children's homes where love and care were in short supply. He talked about his sexuality, and about how he used this as a protection against other kinds of deprivation. He told me how he had vowed to ensure that after these experiences he would never suffer or struggle again. His determination to do this meant that he acquired a great fortune, and sadly went on to abuse others as he himself had been abused.

In telling me all this, Brian was not seeking any gain, other than to offload, and try to make sense of himself. It was probably the first time he was able to be honest with himself, and vulnerable. It was a moment of confession, and I was being his priest and confessor. Brian was clear that he had never had a faith. He also didn't want to seem hypocritical now by hedging his bets in case there was a God whom he was likely to meet in the near future. The tragedy of Brian's life was that he never knew or understood what love means. He mistook it for something which is was most definitely not, and as a consequence he hurt both himself and many others in the process.

I suspect that Brian had many so-called friends when he was a wealthy man living the high life. However, when I took his funeral, there was only one family member attending, out of a sense of duty. It took place on the Isle of Wight, to avoid public scrutiny, and not to bring further shame or attention to family members. I also took a memorial service for Brian in the prison, as is customary. A dozen or so prisoners came. I gave them the opportunity, as I always do, to share their memories of the deceased. They described a generous man, who bought gifts for fellow prisoners whom he called friends, a person of goodwill whom they would remember fondly.

One of the greatest fears of younger prisoners is of having a bereavement whilst they are in prison. Those that come to prison late in life, or those who have been in prison a long time, fear dying in prison.

Prison is a place where most choose not to live, and yet many will live there for a large proportion of their lives. With our increasingly elderly prison population nationally, and the specifics of our client group at HMP Isle of Wight, we were likely to acquire the unfortunate reputation of a place to come to die. One week I was putting up posters advertising memorial services for prisoners who have died, we had two such posters on each wing, and the visual impact as well as the psychological impact on the others in the prison must have been immense.

We are aware of the impact of self-inflicted deaths on other prisoners, but are we also mindful of the impact of deaths generally on the rest of the population? Do prisoners have less hope and motivation to take care of themselves physically in an environment from which they can see no way out? How do you avoid slipping into depression and despair when you arrive in prison in your sixties, seventies or even eighties and are serving long sentences? Or when you are still in a category B prison after twenty years and have been turned down for parole once again? Could the rise in deaths in custody stem not only from an increase in the ageing population, but in the psychological impact of witnessing other prisoners dying in prison?

Another older prisoner told me that he was dying and that there was no further treatment he could be offered for his medical condition. Jim was a proud man, in his eighties, ex-military with a distinguished career. He had newspaper cuttings on the wall of his room with himself with royalty and celebrities involved in various worthy causes.

I first met Jim at a memorial for another of our prisoners. Jim, a man who speaks his mind, told me of his condition, in a matter-of-fact way. A man who has seen action, and has killed people himself whilst on military service, has more awareness of death than many. Jim refused to come to our hospital unit. He had friends on the wing, he held court there, offering the wisdom of his years to any prepared to accept it. He didn't want to go to hospital which was on another site of HMP Isle of Wight—in Albany; he was in Parkhurst. If he had gone there, it would be impossible for him to see any of his friends. Even for residents of Albany, it was difficult to see friends who were patients in the hospital wing. Jim wanted to maintain his independence, such as it was, for as long as he could. His room in our prison was his home, for now, though he hoped that he might be transferred to the mainland to be near his wife and children so that they could visit him more easily. On one occasion Jim nearly died. If it hadn't been for the swift and professional action of prison officers, he would have done. I went to see him following this. Jim was surprised and grateful that I had done so. He was also surprised that the staff had bothered to resuscitate him. He wrote to the governor of the prison as well as to the individuals concerned to thank them. Not a religious man, Jim would say he's seen too much action to believe in much, but a spiritual person nevertheless, clearly searching for meaning and self-worth in his situation. He said that he still has faith and hope in something, for without it he would probably give up. The actions of the staff in saving his life gave him more cause for hope and faith in humanity.

Good enough deaths in a hospice

The hospice is a place with authority where death is regarded as part of the natural order of life itself. There are staff who are experts in the field of palliative care and treatment at the end of life. Most people have only ever experienced one or two deaths in their lives; they may never have seen someone die or been close to a dead person before. On a particular shift, hospice nurses may deal with more deaths than the average person experiences in a lifetime.

When someone comes to the hospice, they are encouraged to express their pain—they are given space to articulate their fears. Fear of what is unknown is very common, so if palliative care staff can describe what death might look like, this can be very helpful. A hospice is a place of great compassion and immense kindness, where nothing is too much trouble; where families are treated with the same respect as the patients; where the smallest details of a person's life are respected and valued.

It is in this context of compassion and kindness, that immense emotional, spiritual and psychological change can take place. Sometimes people are transferred from the hospital or their residential home when their death is imminent. They may only have a matter of a few hours in the hospice, but the patient will be made comfortable, free from pain and enabled to die peacefully. The family may also experience relief knowing that they can spend these last moments in a dignified environment, where they can have privacy and quiet, as well as time and space to say a meaningful farewell, rather than a hurried, awkward and traumatic goodbye.

Do hospice staff expect to see emotional, spiritual, social and physical peace in everyone as they die? Having encountered, in prisons, death which could only be described as "good enough", I was struck by the difference in expectations of dying in a hospice. Certainly, the standard set for dying here is incredibly high. I have heard of a hospice recently whose strapline is that everyone who comes to the hospice will have a pain-free death! To expect every death in a hospice to be pain-free and "good" seems to me to put undue pressure on those who work in it, and on the patients themselves or their families. On some days the staff may have to deal with multiple deaths; this means relating to several grieving families at the same time, as well as dealing with the practicalities of laying out the bodies, contacting funeral directors and cleaning the rooms for the next patient. How realistic is it to hope for a good death for all in these circumstances?

Given that grief and loss are accompanied frequently with anger, I have wondered why there is not more expression of it in the hospice itself. Surely, more people who are dying are angry? I suspect that patients who have had a long illness, or who have experienced several rounds of treatment, have had to deal with their anger elsewhere before coming to the hospice. Perhaps oncology and palliative care consultants and nurses in acute settings are more likely to be on the receiving end of this than hospice staff. Perhaps by even coming to the hospice people are more accepting of the fact that they are dying. I have noticed that when someone dies who does seem angry, some hospice staff feel that they have somehow let them down and wish they could have resolved this pain with them or for them before they died.

The deaths which staff are likely to comment on as having been less peaceful are generally those of younger patients. Perhaps this is when the perception of the injustice of life seems to come to the surface more readily. How can you observe a mother of young children die and not feel her pain as well as knowing the grief that the young children will have to face? A hospice may be able to ease the physical pain, and even the emotional pain for a while, but it cannot change the reality that death and dying can be very cruel.

When a member of staff is confronted by an angry relative—and this is astonishingly rare—it is unfamiliar. Perhaps that is because the ethos of the hospice is to provide care for all the family rather than just the patient. Perhaps there are more resources than in a hospital to ensure that this happens. There are families, of course, where there is tension and dispute; not every family is a happy one, and not every patient is loved by them. Sometimes there is the hope that the circumstances of being with the dying person will bring about reconciliation between warring factions; often this is the wish of the person who is dying. Patients have told me that one of their greatest fears is of leaving the family still quarrelling and not being there to keep the peace. Sometimes the patient will request that certain family members are not permitted to visit or cannot visit when certain others are around. It can be highly complicated for staff to negotiate their way through all of this, without causing upset. While families are sometimes reconciled when someone is dying, this will not always happen, and the best that can be expected is a temporary truce. War may well erupt again in planning the funeral or when the will is read!

The early hospice model was to offer support to patients with cancer. In these circumstances, perhaps, there was a more predictable order of events: receiving a diagnosis; experiencing all the emotions associated with hearing this news; receiving treatment until there was nothing else to be done; then coming to the hospice for their final days, to die peacefully. It is possible that there was an unconscious bias to bring to the hospice people who would be appreciative of the services and who would die a good death. Hospices now are becoming increasingly inclusive. As well as patients having more complex co-morbidities, people may come with a history of addictions, mental health needs, personality disorder, dementia. People who have been homeless or in prison will also come into the hospice with life-limiting conditions and should receive the same level of care. Some patients will have conditions that appear to be related to lifestyle and behavioural choices, and there may be the temptation to regard them differently to patients whose illness is unrelated to their lifestyle.

There will be some patients that certain staff find difficult to care for, either because they remind them of someone close to them who has died; or they are too similar in age or background; or they just can't get along with them. Allowing staff to be individuals is just as important as recognizing the uniqueness of each patient. A wise senior staff member will encourage sharing of roles and organizing shifts to ensure that the member of staff is able to take time away when needed. There is also the possibility of over-identification between staff and patients; so it is important to have good supervision, in order to develop self-awareness and emotional boundaries.

There are many powerful emotions at play when someone is dying; in the patient, and in their relatives. Not everyone is emotionally literate or able to identify or name their feelings at the best of times, let alone at a highly charged time of death. This can mean that emotions are projected onto the staff at the hospice or the organization. A mother, whose young adult daughter died unexpectedly quickly and alone, appeared to express anger that she had not been called in time. Despite knowing that it can often happen that a patient dies alone, and unexpectedly, the staff were concerned that they had done something wrong and were highly self-critical. While it is always important for staff to monitor their actions, it is equally important to recognize that anger is a part of grief, and a mother who has lost a daughter is likely to want to project her anger somewhere. In this particular situation, there was a highly complex relationship between the daughter and mother, and it was likely that the mother felt anger at the daughter for years of suffering she had gone through; there may also have been anger at herself for leaving the hospice and regrets for having done so.

Dying is an emotional minefield, and whilst some people die when they have done the necessary emotional work to do so, others die before they have reached that point. There is then a feeling of work left undone, and unresolved, and intuitively staff sense that it is messier than they would like.

Given the characters of the patients and their individual needs, the complexities of family dynamics, the melting-pot of emotions, the baggage of people's lives, and all the uncertainties surrounding death and beyond, it seems appropriate and realistic to hope for a "good enough" death for most patients in a hospice, hospital or indeed a prison. The fact that many more patients experience a "good death" is testimony to the care and compassion that patients and their families receive, and to the resilience and adaptability of the human spirit in the face of the greatest challenge of our existence, death itself.

Theological reflections

I have used the term "good enough" to consider the experience of people dying in prison and a hospice. It has provided a realistic way of looking at the expectations of others to enable people to die as well as they can, in whatever circumstance they may be. I now turn to the Christian story to see if there are any theological frames of reference for looking at this middle ground.

I go back to the Passion narrative, for it is all about Jesus' impending death and dying. As a preacher I have frequently found it easier to recount the story of the crucifixion than to engage too swiftly with the resurrection. It has at times been difficult to hold on to the resurrection hope and joy and to present it as authentically connected to the human experience. At times Good Friday and Easter Day have seemed to me like polar opposites; too black and white, too far apart, too dualistic to make any pastoral or theological sense.

However, there is a space in between these two momentous events—death and new life—which I am beginning to recognize as helpful, and that is Holy Saturday. This is the day after the crucifixion when Jesus' body is in the tomb, when his spirit descended into hell (according to the Apostles' Creed) and when for the disciples there must have been the numbness and shock of early grief. In the previous chapter I considered the place of Holy Saturday in reflecting theologically on suicide, and I discussed the concept of the Harrowing of Hell.

I now consider the value of Holy Saturday as the liminal space—the place of transition, potential and meaning which is truly sacred. The word "liminal" comes from the Latin word *limen* meaning threshold. It suggests a space between what was, and what may come next. It is a place of transition, waiting and not knowing. Liminal space is where transformation takes place, if we learn to wait and let it form us.

This is the position I hold in pastoral relationships, and in my theological viewpoint. This is a spiritual and emotional limbo, not knowing what may emerge, staying with the situation as it is, not quite in the moment of utter darkness, but standing very close to it. It is a position of ambivalence and uncertainty—not the joyous revelation of Easter morning, or the actual agony of the moment of death, but somewhere in between. This is not a comfortable spiritual home, but it feels very appropriate and real. It feels suitably messy to be genuinely human and yet it contains potential, which feels divine. Maybe it is incarnational mystery? In pastoral terms it is the place which holds the questions of

- What will happen to me next?
- Is there life beyond this existence?
- Does my life have any meaning?

In this Holy Saturday place there is potential, and that gives me hope; but there is no definitive answer, and that makes it authentic. The language in this place is always tentative and suggestive rather than authoritative and dogmatic. I don't know, but I hope; perhaps it is the place of faith, where there is always space for doubt? Maybe I have always inhabited this liminal space, for it feels very familiar and despite it being uncomfortable, it also feels like home. It is possible that because I have spent so long within this context of in between, that people I encounter feel a sense of reassurance when we talk together; for if I can be at ease with uncertainty, then that gives others assurance that it is also acceptable for them to be in this place too, and that we can each be held and supported by one another.

When people who are dying articulate to me the big existential questions, which they often do, even if they do not express them in words, I find myself saying, one day we will know, and it is likely that they will know sooner than I will! It is the wonderful image of 1 Corinthians 13:12: now we see in a mirror dimly, then we shall see face to face; now I know in part, then I shall know in full, even as I am fully known. The Holy Saturday place of theology, pastoral encounter, and spirituality is definitely seeing in a mirror dimly and at times it is so misted over that it isn't possible to see anything at all!

In my pastoral encounters with people on the edge of death, I have been very conscious of this liminal space. It is often silent, but resonant with meaning. There is a lot of waiting here, a lot of uncertainty. There is pain, but also the potential for release. It feels like a tug of war between what is known and what is unknowable. For some people watching alongside those who inhabit this space, it is too painful to remain here, they want to rush back to the familiar, cut the grass, do the shopping—anything which, however trivial, is certain, tangible and practical. Others are able to wait, in the intensity of this liminal space, between having and letting go, between presence and absence, somewhere between the sadness of saying goodbye and the reality of having done so. This is sacred space; this is agony and ambivalence. This is a place of deep meaning, deep emotion, deep experience. On this holy ground it feels as if one should remove one's shoes, bow in reverence, stand in awe. All too soon there will be the practicalities to attend to, the continuing of life to engage with. But in this humbling and privileged waiting space, this Holy Saturday experience, there is a profundity which elevates and enriches the soul.

CHAPTER 6

Dealing with Grief and Bereavement

The British psychiatrist Colin Murray Parkes writes that "[b]ereavement is . . . the most severe life experience that most of us can expect to experience."[5] *In this chapter I consider what is the purpose and normal process of grief. How does it differ for those in prison, and what are the barriers to grieving for prisoners? Using experiences from the hospice I look at the grief of the person who is dying as well as the grief of the bereaved. I reflect on the role and contribution chaplains can make in these circumstances.*

The dying person's grief

As a chaplain working in a hospice, one experiences grief in many facets, forms and stages. Grief is the process of adjustment to loss which the person who is dying deals with daily as they adapt to change in circumstance, loss of function, capacity and control. They face the loss of leaving loved ones behind and the prospect of no longer existing. They also face the loss of their futures, seeing the grandchildren grow, having a foreign holiday, enjoying retirement. As their illness progresses they may face constant change in their abilities, and grieve their loss of identity, role and purpose in life. The person who is dying has a limited time to get to a point of acceptance. Some, of course, won't get there at all and will die when they are still in a state of denial, shock or anger.

Charlie, a man in his forties, was diagnosed with Motor Neurone Disease. Life expectancy following this diagnosis is about two years. In the final stages of the illness, the mind is still active and unimpaired, but the functioning of the body is increasingly limited, until one becomes "locked in". This was the scenario that Charlie was facing. In a very short space of time after being diagnosed he had to move out of the family home and saw less and less of his children. He was housed in a nursing home and went from a socially independent adult in mid-life to being dependent on others and surrounded by people advanced in years. He lost his mobility, and although he acquired an electric wheelchair, his options for getting to places he loved were greatly reduced. He became financially dependent on benefits, as he was unable to work. Charlie's sense of self, which had been shaped by being a father, a lover, a provider, an achiever, was radically challenged. He attended the hospice daycentre weekly, and those of us who saw him recognized further advances of his condition, as he first lost movement of his legs, then his arms. The one thing he was able to do was to talk, but eventually his speech would become impaired and even this would be taken away. All the elements of total pain were apparent in Charlie's situation: social, physical, financial, emotional and spiritual.

When Andy was told that his cancer was untreatable, he embraced the situation with a determination to make the last months of his life fruitful. He went on a spending spree to indulge his interests—bought himself art materials, a new laptop on which he wanted to write a play, a musical instrument. He wanted to do things he had never had time to do before. However, the speed with which his illness advanced meant that the items had barely arrived through the post, before he was admitted to the hospice for end-of-life care. Andy then had to face the loss, not only of his long-term future, but even of his short-term dreams; not surprisingly he felt cheated and angry that even this was taken away from him.

Lena, a woman in her late forties, had been a nurse. She first came to the hospice for symptom control. Her condition made her breathless and she tired easily and yet she had an urgent desire to talk. She had an intellectual understanding of what was happening to her from her professional background and she knew what was likely to happen in the future. She had been told that she probably had a few months to live. The most important thing to her was to renew her marriage vows. In her determination to make this happen, she developed the most complicated plans. At first, she planned to go abroad. She looked up places on the internet and spent hours planning where and when it would take place. She made copious notes on scraps of paper, which she would shuffle around in the drawer of her bedside cabinet. She drew diagrams of the picture she would give to her husband with the vows printed on.

It was a heart-breaking situation to hear Lena talk, barely pausing for breath, and telling me her convoluted ideas, when it seemed so apparent to me that it would be impossible for them to be realized. I sensed that if she stopped talking and planning, the reality of her situation would surface, and she was doing all that she could to keep it away. However, there were moments when she would admit to herself that perhaps she was being too ambitious, and then we could talk about alternative scenarios which might be achievable, like visiting a favourite place nearby with her husband. In the end her condition deteriorated rapidly. She opted for active treatment to extend her life as long as possible, so she was taken to the hospital, and I lost touch with her for a few weeks. Eventually, Lena came back to the hospice. I went to see her. She could no longer speak, and it was clear that she was close to death. She was alone. None of her dreams to renew her wedding vows had been realized. She lay in bed, and wept as I held her hand for some time. She died shortly afterwards.

The grief of the one who is dying can be immense. Some people like Andy and Charlie found it helpful to articulate their feelings and pains, to people like myself and others in the multi-disciplinary hospice team. Others, like Lena, could not face it. Accompanying someone who is experiencing the grief of their own death, one can only travel at their pace, walking alongside them, respecting their wishes and being available to them should they need to talk.

I have recently been introduced by a palliative care consultant to a way of gently encouraging someone to modify their hopes in the face of the reality of their declining health: "wish, worry, wonder". I might have been able to say this to Lena:

> I wish that you were able to go abroad to renew your wedding vows. I wonder whether this is going to be possible? If we look at your health at the moment, I suspect that it would be difficult for you to travel. I wonder, as this is something that really matters to you, whether it might be possible for you to do this somewhere near to home that is special to you both?

Anticipatory grief

The grief of relatives and friends as they watch someone they love die is also enormous. They know the outcome will be the death of the person, and they know that when they have died they will grieve, but as they wait for this inevitability grieving has already started. It is anticipatory grief. They might be imagining life without the person; feeling the anger of dreams that will not now be fulfilled; feeling the panic of how they will manage the finances, or the children; feeling the sadness of facing a permanent farewell.

Families and carers may have been adapting to change, like their relative who is dying, for some considerable time. They may have been taking on new roles and responsibilities as their relative relinquishes them; they may have become carers, have taken on the driving or the finances, or have had to learn to cook. They may have had some time anticipating a loss that is permanent or it may have arisen suddenly and unexpectedly. Anticipatory grieving may or may not affect the process of grief which follows death.

Colin Murray Parkes talks of deprivation associated with the loss of a loved one: the absence of the deceased may bring financial deprivation; deprivation of company or sexual relations; deprivation of emotional or practical support. As a relative, especially a partner, waits for the death of their companion, all these concerns and anxieties may be passing through their minds. If the person who is dying can talk with their families about what is happening and about the impact of their death on those remaining, then some of these deprivations might be minimized, if not avoided altogether. There is a strong emphasis within the hospice movement to encourage people to be financially, practically and emotionally prepared for death well in advance, not leaving it until the last moments of life, when it may be too late.

Simon knew that his wife Alice was dying. They travelled through the stages of grief together by talking honestly and openly. They were able to discuss their finances, her wishes for the funeral, her hopes for his future. They discussed whether or not he should move away; whether he should remarry; they even talked of the designs for a new kitchen, which she would never see, but which it gave her pleasure to think about. Simon grieved when she died. But he was also able to experience joy and peace when she did. The fact that they had been able to talk about important things meant that he knew she accepted dying, and that gave him comfort. Because they had talked, Simon knew what Alice's wishes were, so that he didn't have to agonize over the choices he made afterwards—to change the kitchen, and to remarry. By being able to engage in this way together, Alice felt that she had ended her life well by giving advice, guidance and permissions to her husband who was her greatest concern as she died, and it meant that the deprivations of loss that Simon would feel after her death were reduced.

Sometimes other family members and friends are surprised when a bereaved partner appears to move on quickly after the death of a loved one. They might be angry or disapproving of them and feel that it shows disrespect to the one who has died. However, it could be the case that, like Simon and Alice, the couple have talked about and prepared for the reality of death, so that they have both been more peaceful when it has happened. They may have both experienced the anticipatory grief of ending together and done much of the hard work of grief before it has happened, so that the process afterwards for the partner who remains is less arduous.

The journey of grief

It is a massive adjustment facing bereavement and dealing with grief, and the pain it generates is not dissimilar to the total pain of the person who is dying; for there is often physical pain—loss of sleep, feeling sick or being unable to eat, exhaustion; emotional pain—mood swings, anger, depression, lack of motivation; social pain—loneliness, not wanting to be a burden, isolation; spiritual pain—not knowing who I am any more, does my life have any meaning, loss of purpose and hope.

Death, even when it is expected, anticipated or welcomed as a release, is accompanied by grief. Even if grief has been experienced before, it is different each time. It will be different depending on the circumstances of death, the relationship and attachment to the person who has died, the previous experiences of death, and how each death is perceived. However much one has thought about death or experienced it as a professional person, no one can know exactly how they will react or deal with the death of someone they are closest to. Grief always takes us into uncharted emotional territory which is exhausting as well as unfamiliar.

The stages of grief are well documented and understood. Elizabeth Kübler-Ross describes patients who are facing death as experiencing shock, denial, anger, bargaining and acceptance. Colin Murray Parkes identifies similar stages of grief. While grief is widely understood as a process, it is not linear, not everyone experiences every stage, and the movement from one phase to another and back again can be very rapid.

It can be immensely helpful for people who are grieving to learn that grief is a process, and that what they may be feeling is "normal". I often explain this to people; letting them know that mood swings and the utter exhaustion which accompanies them is to be expected gives them permission to accept what they are feeling, and not to judge themselves for wanting it to be over. Grief can feel anything but normal when you are living through it. It is unpredictable; one moment you can feel you are coping and the next you are in floods of tears; it can be triggered by the smallest act, piece of music, smell. It has no end, just variations on a theme.

I had been in ordained ministry for eighteen years when my father died. I had dealt with many people who had had bereavements in that time. I had read widely about grief. In the early days of grieving I was very self-critical, because I felt that it was only when I experienced grief at first hand that I really understood what it was like. I felt that my ministry with the bereaved previously had been academic only, ineffectual and a sham, because until I went through it myself, in the way that I did, I had had no idea what I was talking about. It was perhaps an extreme response, but there is a fundamental difference between knowledge that is understood, and the wisdom that comes through personal experience.

No two people experience grief in the same way. Parents of a young man in the hospice expressed their sorrow very differently when he died; the father was matter of fact and business-like. He did not want to talk about anything, he had barely wanted to stay at his son's bedside as he was dying. He didn't cry. The mother had cradled her son's head as he was dying and told him of all the wonderful things he had done in his life and all he had meant to her. She wept and needed to talk. She came into the chapel and told me exactly what had happened a few minutes before. Although she was very emotional, she said she was peaceful too; her son was not suffering any more. She also described a great calm that had come over her as he died. She described smells in the room which she noticed at that moment; one was pipe tobacco and the other violets. She associated these smells with her own father who had died and her older sister who had died as a young child. She took great comfort from this, believing that her deceased relatives whom she cared about had come to meet her son and that she was handing him over to them.

In a hospice, families of patients are surrounded by people who care, by many who are going through the same kind of experience and pain, and they describe feeling at home, and safe. Here it is accepted that you will be emotional, that you may need to talk or ask questions, and there are people to listen and answer, it is understood that you may want to be on your own. Here death is not taboo, it is seen as a normal part of life. Families may be there for a few hours, or for a few weeks, but it can quickly feel like a second home. It can be very hard for some families when their relative dies because they feel they no longer have the right to come to the hospice. They feel they will be intruding if they do appear, as the staff will be busy with the next patient who has replaced their loved one. Strong attachments are formed between the families and the staff, and to some it can feel like another rejection, another grief, to let go of the hospice. I frequently hear of relatives saying they want to volunteer, to give something back to the hospice. I wonder whether they are wanting a legitimate reason to come back to the hospice and feel a sense of belonging, acceptance and comfort again.

In much of the rest of the world and life, a grieving person can feel like an anomaly, someone who makes people feel uncomfortable, as they don't really know how to react or what to say. A person who is grieving doesn't really know how they fit in "normal life" any more. If they have been in a relationship where they have done everything together, do they continue to attend things on their own? Will they drag the mood of a social event down if they go along? How often can they talk about their loved one before friends start to get bored and their eyes glaze over? People who have been bereaved describe situations when people have deliberately avoided speaking to them, or crossed the road to avoid them, rather than talking to them. They can be left feeling hurt and disappointed in friends and neighbours whom they had thought would be more understanding of their situation.

A hospice can provide a sanctuary for someone negotiating their way through grief. For some it is a place to retreat to, a place of welcome and familiarity, where people can feel close to the person who has died there, or amongst friends or people who have supported them. Activities in the hospice, like the café, or the community choir, can give someone who is grieving a legitimate reason to come there and meet others who may well understand what they are going through. It is probably slightly easier to come to a social event at the hospice when you have been bereaved, than to go to a theatre or a café on your own. There will be specific bereavement support available, for individuals or as part of a group. There may be art and music therapy or drama on offer, for adults or children. There are also specific support groups for families where there has been a suicide. This can really help to reduce the sense of isolation and feeling the odd one out in the rest of the world. In a hospice there will always be someone to talk to, and others who have travelled the road of grief too, and who are able to encourage you when you need it. There are also regular memorial services, as well as large annual events of remembrance, to bring together people who have experienced loss.

Complicated grief

If grieving is hard work when a death is expected and has been prepared for, how much more difficult will grief be when it is a sudden death, a violent death, a death by murder, a death by suicide? Grief in these situations is complicated and can be accompanied by secrecy and shame. Griefs associated with motherhood are frequently hidden and unspoken; women who have had abortions often carry guilt and may have difficulty forgiving themselves and moving on from this experience. I met many women in prison who have also carried this pain, and who have masked their feelings with drugs or alcohol, or others who already had addictions and felt unable to keep the child because of their lifestyles.

I was asked to see a young woman from Jamaica, Charlene, who had recently come to HMP Downview sentenced to several years' imprisonment for drug importation. The staff were concerned that she was increasingly withdrawn and would barely speak to anyone. I brought her to my office and invited her to talk, if she wanted to, about what was troubling her. After establishing a rapport, she eventually told me in as few words as possible, and without making eye contact, that she had had an abortion. It transpired that at the airport she had been required to be X-rayed because of the drugs found in her person. She discovered later that she was pregnant. She was advised that because of the amount of radiation she had been exposed to, the baby she was carrying was at risk, and she was advised to consider a termination. As she was also facing a sentence of several years, this was an additional factor in her decision. It had clearly been a very traumatic time for her, and she had felt very ambivalent about it, leaving the final decision to go ahead with the abortion until the last moment.

By the time Charlene spoke to me, she had had several weeks since the abortion and was deeply troubled by the decision she had made and wracked with guilt at having made it. She was also distressed by the fact that she had never held the baby and chose not to see it or to discover what sex the baby was. She was a tormented soul, grieving for an unknown child, whom she felt she had killed. I felt that she had had no closure and that if this were possible she might be able to find some peace. Holding out little hope, I contacted the chaplain at the hospital where the abortion had taken place. She was extremely helpful and looked into the situation for me. It transpired that because Charlene had been so ambivalent about her decision, the staff had kept the baby's body just in case. They were able to tell us what the sex was, and so Charlene was able to name her. Working together, the prison, the hospital and the funeral directors enabled Charlene to attend her daughter's funeral, which I conducted, and the child was buried with dignity and many tears. Charlene was then able to grieve for her daughter and move on with her life.

Women who have had children taken into care or have given up their children for adoption also experience complex grief and guilt. In Holloway I supported women who have had to make this decision, and I was present when a mother had a final visit with her child before he was adopted. I also met elderly women who have had this kind of experience and who have lived with the secret all their lives, keeping if from their husbands and subsequent children. There were also women who had been adopted, and there was loss for them too as they wrestled with the questions of why their natural mothers could not keep them.

Loss from miscarriage or stillbirth is also complicated; although it is much more widely and sensitively acknowledged now, it has not been always so. Women who have experienced loss like this may have carried the pain of this grief for years, and even if they have had children later, they do not replace the children who have been lost. The bond between mother and baby starts early in pregnancy, and grief about the death of an unborn child may reflect this bond, but the grief is also for the future which has been anticipated and cannot now be realized.

I met prisoners, men and women, who had killed their partner, friend or close relative, including their children, often in situations of domestic chaos. They will be in prison facing the charge of murder, and yet they are also grieving for the person they have killed.

The tragedy of these circumstances is compounded by abuse which may well have been present and prevalent. Then the partner left has to come to terms with the loss of someone they have loved, but in healing that they may also begin to acknowledge—perhaps for the first time—the abuse that they have experienced. Then they may grieve again for the lost relationship they wished they had had or feel regret that they had not sought help or left the relationship sooner.

These kinds of situations are extremely emotionally complicated, and may only be unravelled after many years of therapeutic input. As a chaplain I have been asked to say prayers or light candles for someone by the person who has killed them. I have taken prisoners to chapel at the time of the deceased person's funeral, for of course, it would be entirely inappropriate for the prisoner to attend. Holding on to the belief that God is in the mess and muddle of life and understands its complexities better than I can hope to do, has enabled me to do or say something which is meaningful in this kind of situation.

Coping with bereavement in prison

Those who experience a bereavement whilst in prison have to deal with the loss of a loved one without the comfort and support of being with family or friends. There will be no one around who has known the deceased, so there will be no one that the prisoner can share their memories with. It is very unlikely that they will have been with the relative at the time of death, and they may not have seen them for a considerable time. Some prisoners are given compassionate leave if the relative is a very close blood relative, to see them for a short visit before they die or to attend the funeral afterwards. It is an invidious choice that they must make. Do I want to see my relative in hospital accompanied by prison staff and handcuffed to them? Or do I want to attend the funeral in the same way and be subject to the scrutiny and comments of all the family and friends at once? Which will bring less shame to the family and the dying or deceased? Which will bring me any closure?

Even if a prisoner may wish to, they may not even be able to go to the funeral; it will depend on the security department's assessment of the situation, based on the closeness of the relationship to the prisoner, the feasibility of making the journey, and whether or not the family want them there. If the family do want the prisoner to attend, they will have to prove the closeness of the relationship, finding birth certificates for parents, or children, or evidence to show that a grandparent brought them up. So there may be no closure for the prisoner and the grieving process may be very difficult as a consequence. There have been foreign national prisoners whose relatives have died in their home countries, so there is no chance that they can be present at the funeral. All we as staff and chaplains could do for the prisoner was to provide a listening ear, offer them some space in which to grieve and give them the opportunity to come to the chapel and say prayers or light a candle.

There is very little psychological support for dealing with bereavement in prison. There are few if any counsellors; some prisons will have access to Cruse bereavement counselling volunteers, but even here the demand will outweigh the supply, and although this organization does fantastic work, the complexity of grief for prisoners suggests that specialist support would be more appropriate. Often it falls to the chaplains to offer pastoral listening and compassionate care.

People in prison who experience a death of a relative are likely to feel regret and guilt more than most. Some will relate the loss of their loved one directly to the fact that they are in prison. "If I had not come to prison, they would never have died." "The stress of my being here caused my parent to have a heart attack." Alongside the inevitable "if onlys" when bereaved, there are the additional "if onlys" of imprisonment, and together they can seem overwhelming. For many people, coming to prison itself is a grief-generating experience since it involves so many losses—of freedom, home, job, family, control, and even of hope. Even if the individual has come to terms with the losses of being in prison, the feelings of despair and sadness can be reawakened quickly by an additional loss of a family member.

I met many prisoners who had experienced loss at an early age, either through abandonment as children, being taken into care, or the death of a significant stable figure at a formative stage. Losses like these, without appropriate support and understanding, may have triggered depression, self-harm, educational or behavioural problems, criminal activity, promiscuity or addictions. Many prisoners had unresolved griefs before coming to prison, which an additional bereavement complicates further. If prisoners have suppressed or masked the pain of loss previously through drugs or alcohol, they have few coping strategies and little emotional resilience to cope with an additional loss without these crutches. I found this particularly the case when working with women in prison; the risk of self-harm or suicide could be greatly increased when a female prisoner was bereaved again.

Often other prisoners were able to offer comfort and support to one another. They will probably not have known the deceased, but they may be familiar with loss and grief themselves, outside prison or within it. This kind of support may come informally from prisoners on the wing, or through the Prison Listener Scheme—prisoners who are trained by the Samaritans, to provide a listening service at any time of the day or night. You can never measure what does not happen, but I am sure that Prison Listeners have been able to save many lives of prisoners who, when faced with a bereavement in the family, would otherwise have sought to kill themselves.

Breaking bad news

One of the tasks of the chaplain in the prison is to inform a prisoner when there has been a death in their family. When a phone call is received about a death, a chaplain, or another member of staff, must check the information with the police, a hospital or coroner. It is not sufficient to accept the word of a relative as there have been occasions when false information has been given for some other gain. It can be hard for families to understand why we need to check what they are saying as it is painful enough to experience a loss, without then feeling you are not believed. Once the death has been formally confirmed by an external source, and sometimes this can take some considerable time, a chaplain is required to visit the prisoner concerned and tell them of the death. There have been innumerable times when I have had to do this; it is one of the most challenging tasks of the role.

Prisoners often said that they found it hard to believe that a relative had really died. Anyone who is bereaved takes time to adjust and may be in shock so it is hard to take in what has happened. For a person in prison that sense of unreality may last a long time, as they cannot have the experiences that will make the loss more real: like visiting places with which the deceased is associated. Sometimes, I suspect, it is only after the prisoner has been released that reality really sinks in, and the process of grief can begin.

I have had to inform prisoners of the death of their closest relatives—parents, grandparents, siblings. I have had to tell prisoners that their children have died. All these have been traumatic and tragic, and frequently I have felt inadequate and helpless. On one occasion I had to inform a prisoner that all her immediate family had been killed in a plane crash in Nigeria. The young woman was in such shock that she did not speak for several days, and she refused to eat; she lay on her bed and literally turned her face to the wall. I sat with her in her cell for long periods. I simply sat and shared her painful silence. There was nothing that could be said to alleviate her sorrow. Eventually she began to emerge from the depths of her sorrow and slowly began to engage in activity again. She was due to be repatriated a few weeks later, and on the day of her removal to a detention centre, she came to the chapel with a friend.

She wanted to say goodbye and asked me to pray with her. She knelt in front of me as a gesture of respect which was traditional in her culture and thanked me for all I had done for her. I could not bear to see her express such gratitude in this way when I had done so little. I knelt alongside her, and we both shed tears together of the journey of sorrow we had shared. I will never know how she fared once she returned home.

Not all loss is as extreme as this, but every grief is painful and when preparing to tell someone of a death of a relative you never know how they will react. It is always necessary to inform prison staff that you are about to break some bad news and to ask for their presence and support so that they can assist as necessary. Having worked first with women in prison, who generally express their emotions easily, I was taken aback the first time I went to tell a male prisoner that his mother had died. He was matter of fact, unemotional, and barely asked any questions or needed any support. I had to ask him a few times if he was all right, as I had never before experienced so little reaction or response. In contrast, I have informed a young woman whose grandmother died, who sat on the floor in a curled-up position and refused to be moved. I have informed a woman from West Africa that her mother had died, and she wailed loudly and beat her head against the floor. Understanding that there may be cultural and gender differences in the way that grief is expressed is important.

Caring for the grieving

It is essential to understand the process and pains of grief when offering support to someone who is bereaved. C. S. Lewis, writing after his wife died, was surprised that the physical sensations of grief were so similar to those associated with fear—fluttering stomach, restlessness, yawning.[6] Grief can also feel like anxiety or depression and some bereaved people will feel suicidal, so being aware of the range and depth of emotions is vital if the pastor is to care effectively. Given how isolated and alone people who have been bereaved can feel, listening to them is paramount.

As soon as I saw my husband shortly after my father died, I wanted to tell him about what had happened in detail. It seemed essential to me to describe the experience to someone who would simply listen. The intensity of the time I spent with my father in his last hours means that I can recall clearly those hours more clearly than any other 24 hours in my life. I have noticed this same need in others to tell the narrative of the moment of death to someone. Therefore I always invite people to do so when I meet with them to discuss a funeral, and I frequently find that people who have been bereaved for a long time also want to share this part of their loss in a pastoral conversation. Perhaps there are not many people in everyday life who are willing to listen to this aspect of someone's experience.

The intensity of accompanying someone who is dying increases awareness and sensitivity to what is happening around you. It is not until after the event that you realize that you can describe in detail sounds, smells and sights of that moment and the words and actions of others. If we are meant to live fully in the moment, fully aware and focused on now, then it is probably when witnessing someone dying that we are most alive! Perhaps because we are focused on being there, with another person, our minds are stilled from all the planning and distractions of thought that usually assail us, and we are more attuned to our emotions, and our physical responses to them, than at most other occasions. It is perhaps because of the emotional intensity of the situation that the bereaved person may need to recount the details many times in order to process the experience more effectively.

As someone tells the story of the death of a loved one, you can also hear more about their emotional state and aspects of their loss which might need to be revisited. You can identify whether it has been traumatic for them and whether they have been disturbed by what they have witnessed. You can hear anger or acceptance in their tone. There might be regrets for things said or not said, or guilt for not being there when they felt they should. You can pick up tensions in the family, if one member has been present and another has not, or when one has dominated or another not pulled their weight. You can pick up where they are placed in the journey of grief, if they are in denial, in shock, or angry, or if it is just all too overwhelming and they cannot yet say anything. It is so important to listen at every level to what is said and not said, to read body language and symbols; to let someone express themselves at their own pace and allow them plenty of time, and to accept without judgement whatever they say.

I find people who have been bereaved can feel totally out of their depth, and in such unfamiliar emotional territory that they feel they are going mad. Acknowledging to them the enormity of grief, how hard it is, and the normality of the seemingly abnormal can be helpful. Grief is unpredictable and a long process. Sometimes people think that because they have had a better day that they are "over it" only to discover that the next day they are struggling with despair and despondency again. Sometimes they feel that the expectations of others are a burden and that people think they should be behaving like this or they should be doing that. Sometimes they find they are at odds with others in their family who are grieving differently, and they cannot talk to those that are around them. It is astounding how many people who have never experienced a significant loss are apparently experts on grief! For someone who has been bereaved, it can be a lifeline to find someone who will listen attentively; who will let them express whatever is going on for them at that moment; not hurry them along in their grief; let them talk about the moment of death or the person who has died for as long as they need.

The one who listens to a bereaved person holds and contains all that they want to express and in doing so can help them feel less isolated. It may be a short-lived feeling, but in that moment of sharing and being heard, they can feel some comfort. Hopefully they will be able to return to that encounter, long after it has passed, and it will remind them that there are others who are not overwhelmed by their sorrow and who hold a strong belief in their ability to navigate their way through the experience of loss and grief, and who are holding on to this hope for them. As Colin Murray Parkes says of grief:

> In many respects, then, grief can be regarded as an illness. But it can also bring strength. Just as broken bones may end up stronger than unbroken ones, so the experience of grieving can strengthen and bring maturity to those who have previously been protected from misfortune. The pain of grief is just as much part of life as the joy of love; it is, perhaps, the price we pay for love, the cost of commitment.[7]

In many cultures grief is not an individual experience but one that is embraced by the community. In modern Western society this is less so. The concept of mourning, when friends and neighbours offer practical as well as emotional support to the bereaved person for a given period, has been largely lost. Grief is experienced as a private matter which is very individualized. People generally are less comfortable with public expressions of grief and sorrow, and are more inclined to encourage a bereaved person to move on quickly to seeing the positives of what someone has left behind, rather than dwelling on the pains of their absence. Many bereaved people can find comfort in being with others who have also been bereaved, recognizing that they are going through similar experiences to themselves. Pastoral care may be to help someone who is feeling alone with their grief to find other networks, groups and communities for support.

Theological reflection on grief

In the story of the Passion we can see multiple expressions of grief and loss; grief of Jesus as he faces his own death; the anticipatory grief of the disciples as they accompany him in his final hours; the different reactions of those who wait or cannot wait with Jesus as he dies; the varying responses of grief to Jesus' death.

In the final discourse in John's Gospel, Jesus' primary concern is for those he will be leaving.

> A little while, and you will no longer see me, and again a little while, and you will see me . . . Very truly, I tell you, you will weep and mourn, but the world will rejoice; you will have pain, but your pain will turn into joy.
>
> *John 16:16, 20*

Like many people who are facing their own death, Jesus is trying to prepare those around him for the reality of what is to come and the pain of the grief they will feel. Like many family and friends who accompany a dying person, they are not ready or able to face this kind of preparation and conversation, and don't really understand what is being said to them. Jesus recognizes their limitations as well as the emotional pain they now feel.

> I still have many things to say to you, but you cannot bear them now.
>
> *John 16:12*

The loneliness of dying and the desolation of Jesus' grief as he faces his death comes across strongly.

> The hour is coming, indeed it has come, when you will be scattered, each one to his home, and you will leave me alone.
>
> *John 16:32*

Although Jesus later acknowledges that he is not alone, for the Father is with him, the feeling of abandonment by his friends is powerful. In the Garden of Gethsemane this is described most vividly. Here Jesus, like many on the brink of death, is vulnerable, needy, lonely and frightened, begging for this suffering to be over, needing the companionship of his closest friends for support. In the Passion, we see the complete humanity of Jesus.

> He took with him Peter and James and John, and began to be distressed and agitated. And he said to them, "I am deeply grieved, even to death; remain here and keep awake." And going a little farther, he threw himself on the ground and prayed that, if it were possible, the hour might pass from him. He said, "Abba, Father, for you all things are possible; remove this cup from me."
>
> *Mark 14:33–36a*

Throughout the Passion story, there are many layers of pain that Jesus experiences; physical, social, emotional and spiritual; this is the total pain of dying. As readers of the Passion, we tend to hurry quickly on from these passages, to hear the point of acceptance, hope and faith that

Jesus also expresses, for we may feel more comfortable here, than in the reality of Jesus' grief.

> [y]et, not what I want, but what you want.
>
> *Mark 14:36b*

The written text implies that Jesus moves swiftly through the stages of grief to acceptance. However, the emotional torment in the garden is anything but swift, as the vigil on Maundy Thursday night attempts to recreate liturgically.

For the one who is dying, who faces the desolation of death, there may be greater comfort from recognizing that even Jesus, who had the greatest faith in God of anyone, struggled to come to terms with his death, and that even in the moment of his dying cries out with a loud voice:

> My God, my God, why have you forsaken me?
>
> *Mark 15:34*

I shared my reflections of Jesus' experiences in the Garden of Gethsemane with an elderly woman, Evie, in a nursing home. I first met her when she was in the hospice preparing to die. She had been at ease with her impending death. However, she had rallied, gone home, fallen, and then been taken into care. I saw her on a few occasions and took her Communion. On one visit she acknowledged to me that she was confused and anxious. The peace she had previously, had evaporated as she now faced a life of passivity, uncertainty and loneliness in the home where she was living. She was experiencing deep emotional and spiritual distress as she wondered whether her life had any meaning and value any more. She felt that she would never walk again and that the remaining life she had would be one of dependence on others. She was finding this hard to bear, and longed for God to let her die. Her strong faith was wavering.

As I listened attentively to Evie's distress and grief, I was reminded again of W. H. Vanstone's book *The Stature of Waiting* in which he describes the change from Jesus's active ministry to the passivity of the last week of his life. I shared my reflections with Evie and we read the story of the Garden of Gethsemane together, pausing to consider how

Jesus' experiences mirrored Evie's own struggles. It was a moment of revelation for her, as the words and stories that she had heard so often seemed to come alive through her own experience. She began to see how her own suffering was drawing her into a deeper understanding of the pain that Jesus himself experienced and that if she were able to find this profound connection then her own experience of suffering would be transformed. The time that she had left to live was not a waste but an opportunity to discover spiritual insights that would take her deeper into the heart of God.

Evie recognized that her whole perspective on her situation had been changed by this conversation. Both of us were utterly surprised, awed and moved by the revelations of this encounter. As we received Holy Communion together, the significance of this sacrament touched us both. We concluded by singing the wonderful hymn "Just as I am"; the words seemed incredibly poignant. Both Evie and I sensed the presence of God and the guiding of the Holy Spirit which impacted on us greatly. I told Evie that I was writing a book about my reflections and that I would share this experience in it. She was delighted to think that she might be able to help someone else; another way of finding meaning in her own pain.

As well as revealing the grief of Jesus as he faces his own death, the Passion highlights the grief of his friends as they anticipate it. Jesus knows that he is going to die, but his followers find it hard to accept it. The repetition in the final discourse by Jesus, telling them that he will be leaving them soon, suggests that they need to hear it repeatedly in order to grasp it. In Mark's account, at the Last Supper when Jesus predicts that they will all desert him, Peter vehemently denies that he would ever do this, and yet a few hours later he fails to live up to his promise. Peter and the others cannot even stay awake to provide Jesus with companionship when he needs it most, and when Jesus is arrested we are told: "All of them deserted him and fled" (Mark 14:50).

It is very hard for loved ones to stay with someone who is dying. The process of death can be very unpleasant to witness, like a crucifixion—with people struggling to breathe, or being sick, or with bodily distortions due to cancerous growths. Some will remain alongside, others will keep at some distance, others cannot bear to come at all. Many of the followers of Jesus, who loved him dearly, were unable to stay with him. They ran away;

perhaps for fear for their own safety; or because the pain of witnessing another's pain was too great. At the crucifixion itself, in Luke's account, we are told that Jesus' followers, including the women who had accompanied Jesus, "stood at a distance, watching these things" (Luke 23:49). However, in John's account, we are told that the beloved disciple, Jesus' mother, and some of the other women were at the foot of the cross right to the end.

There is often trauma when accompanying someone to death, and for all of those who were able to witness the crucifixion, as well as those who were not, there was unbearable grief to face. There was the tangible grief of losing someone close; there was the trauma of witnessing the horrendous manner of death; and there was also the grief of hopes destroyed, as the disciples' view of Jesus as the Saviour, or Redeemer, were shattered.

Joseph of Arimathea found an outlet for his grief in a practical way, through offering to take care of Jesus' body, and providing the tomb to lay him in. The women similarly responded with activity; seeking to honour Jesus by anointing his body. Many of the other followers retreated and locked themselves away, huddled together for solace and comfort. They were frightened and anxious. Cleopas and his companion just wanted to be home, away from the scenes of horror and away from the overwhelming grief of the group. The walked back to Emmaus. All sought their own way to process and deal with the tragedy and shock of their experiences.

All those who followed Jesus in his ministry, after the events of Good Friday, were left with the most complicated grief to bear. The one they loved had been killed in such a traumatic and humiliating way, and their whole sense of meaning and purpose had been destroyed. Seeing the crucifixion, not from the point of knowing about the resurrection, but from the perspective of those who were present, and recognizing the trauma of their grief and the different ways in which they express it, may have resonance and meaning for those who are currently living with grief and bereavement.

In the gospel story there is a transformation of the sorrow of loss into the joy of resurrection, on the third day. There may be new life after a death for a bereaved person, but it will only be after they have travelled along the arduous journey of grief, a journey which cannot be hurried and which will vary according to each person who experiences it.

CHAPTER 7

Rituals of Dying and Remembering

In this chapter I consider the purpose, meaning and significance of rituals at the end of life. I discuss the value of preparing funerals with those who are dying or their families, and I describe personal experiences of taking funerals for those who are unloved and those who have died by suicide. I reflect on the rituals of Jesus' dying and death and consider whether rituals, and those who conduct them, provide assurance for those standing on a threshold.

Rituals are part of everyone's lives. Sometimes they are associated with traditions or faiths; sometimes they are connected to superstitions; frequently they help us find a sense of identity or belonging. Generally, they shape and give structure to our lives. The need for ritual is greatest, perhaps, at times of change and challenge. They may be the things that we cling to when everything around us is unfamiliar and frightening.

Preparing a funeral with the person who is dying

Some people find comfort as they face their death by preparing their own funeral. It is something over which they feel they have some control when so much else is out of their control. Some will want to write their own eulogy, others will only want to say where they want to be buried or cremated and will leave the rest of the decision making to others.

There are people who take great pains to plan every fine detail of the arrangements. One woman, in her early fifties, asked to make an appointment with me. Linda had already spoken at length to the funeral directors who had alerted me to her wish to sort out who would do her funeral. When I spoke to her, she had pretty much everything worked out and was enjoying finalizing all the arrangements. She had chosen music, readings, venue, and caterers for the wake afterwards. She had even specified what she wanted people to wear: bright colours and red bow ties for the funeral directors! She wanted to go out with a bang and not a whimper! She had clearly informed many of her friends, of whom there was a constant stream into the hospice, of her plans. I met her in the day-centre with a friend, and Linda introduced me to her as the one who would be taking her funeral. The friend, who knew of the funeral arrangements and the party afterwards, said, "We are really looking forward to it!"

Fortunately, we were all able to laugh. Linda's incredibly positive approach to her death was unusual, and I am certain that in dying as she did, she taught the many friends and associates she had on social media, that death need not be feared but can be embraced enthusiastically. She said to me, "I am living more fully than ever before now that I am dying." I told her she was acquiring much wisdom in doing so, and that I would include what she had said in this book to help others.

Another patient, Don, also in his fifties, resisted all conversation about dying. He was dying too soon and was angry about not having time to enjoy his home and retirement with his wife. His wife, who wanted to make his last days positive and happy, feared to talk about his funeral wishes, because it would upset him, or her, or both of them. She asked if I could help. Over the days Don and I talked about all sorts of things, including the prison where we had both worked and known each other previously. On one occasion when I visited him, Don was on his own; he was very sleepy, but he said: "We need to have an important conversation now."

Recognizing the inevitability of death and that it was approaching soon, he had decided he wanted to let me know his wishes. I sat with him for some time. He would make a statement about an item that he cared about and who he wanted to leave it to, and then fall asleep. Then when he awoke after a few minutes, he asked me if I would take his funeral. It is always very humbling when a patient or their family asks me to do this for them. I feel that this is the greatest compliment they could give me about the relationship we have formed. Often it has little to do with a shared belief, or denomination, but is purely because of the relationship we have established. We continued in this staccato kind of conversation, which was immensely important to him, until he had expressed all he wanted to. I wrote his wishes down and relayed them back to him, signed and dated the paper and left it on the table in case he should think of anything else later that mattered to him. I knew that his wife would be visiting and would see the evidence of what we had discussed. After Don died, I was able to sit with his wife and finalize the details of his funeral together; knowing that she was carrying out his wishes was a comfort to her in her grief.

Preparing a funeral with a relative

When a relative asks me to take someone's funeral, I arrange to meet with the family to discuss it with them. If the person had died in the hospice, I am aware that families may have mixed feelings about coming back to the building so soon after the death. If I meet the family at home, it may give me a fuller picture of the deceased and their lives as part of a family unit. If the visit takes place in the home of the deceased, then I will see the home that meant a lot to them, the photos of the people who have mattered to them, the evidence of the hobbies and interests they have had, and I will meet their pets! If I am on the home territory of the family, I think they will be more at ease, and as a guest I am making myself less of an expert in funeral arranging and more of a companion and friend who is genuinely interested in their loved ones and their lives.

There is no formula for these conversations; they are organic and responsive to the situation and the needs of those who are grieving. In the course of the conversation, however, there are some elements which I will ensure are covered: the narrative of the moment of death, awareness of the life of the deceased, their beliefs and their wishes; about the funeral; the wishes and beliefs of the family; who is likely to be attending the funeral, and if they want to take part. I will make sure they are aware of the time constraints of the service if it takes place in the crematorium and ensure that any contributions to eulogies or music are realistically timed.

I will always ask permission to write notes as we talk. I try to include things that the family say verbatim, as this can give the sermon or talk more authenticity in the service. I offer to draw up a structure of the service and will email this to the family as soon as I can. I have learned from experience that doing this quickly can alleviate anxiety in relatives. If I have been delayed in sending this to the family, it has caused unnecessary worry at a time when life for them is already hard enough. I make sure that I allow plenty of time for the visit and make that clear in setting it up and on arrival. I have conducted visits lasting any time between an hour and three hours, depending on the emotional needs of the person I am meeting.

As a chaplain who may have met the deceased in the hospice, and as someone who can spend a significant time with the family afterwards, I am like a bridge between the deceased and the bereaved; the hospice and the home. When the family are visiting someone in the hospice, they have access to all sorts of professionals and support. Once they leave after the death, they may feel quite isolated. They will have to visit the registrar and the funeral director to make arrangements, but these will be more task-focused rather than therapeutic. They may not have been able to talk to anyone about the death or their feelings, except with people who are emotionally involved themselves. Someone in my position is neutral and they can express their feelings without concern for mine. I have frequently found a change in the person as the visit has progressed. They may be heavy-hearted and sorrowful as we begin, but towards the end they look and seem brighter. They find that they have been able to smile and even laugh at some of the memories and stories they have shared, and it gives them a glimmer of realization that the person they love will never be lost to them as long as they can recall them and talk about them. I can also offer reassurance to them about the process of grieving.

What kind of a funeral?

The funeral can be an important ritual for the bereaved. When the deceased has stated that they do not want any ceremony to mark their death, it can be difficult for the family left behind. They may be torn—wanting to respect the wishes of their relative, but recognizing their own need to publicly acknowledge their loss. This raises the question as to who the funeral is for? Is it for the deceased to be able to get a final message out there, or is it part of the grieving process for the family?

Mark had made his wishes known to the funeral director months before coming to the hospice. He was adamant that he didn't want anything to happen, just that he would be buried in a woodland cemetery close to the grave of his mother. His sole relative, a cousin with whom he had kept in touch, felt uncomfortable about doing nothing, as she felt his life had meant more to her, and to a handful of others who wanted to mark the occasion, than he supposed. I suspect that had Mark written his wishes a few weeks after being with us in the hospice, his wishes might have been slightly less stark and bleak. As Mark and I had shared a love of classical music, I was able to tell his cousin that he loved Bach's Cello Suites, and so on a lovely sunny day, a few of us gathered as Mark's cousin said a few words, and his body was placed in the ground to the strains of Bach. Some of us then threw handfuls of earth into the grave and said our goodbyes. It was very touching and dignified, and seemed to keep the balance between the views of the deceased and the needs of the family.

Victor had worked in the funeral industry. He had insisted to his family that he did not want them to go to the crematorium and have a public service for him. Victor's wife and children were ambivalent. They felt the need to do something. It was arranged that I would conduct a private ceremony of farewell to Victor in the chapel of rest at the funeral directors, and then I and his colleagues from the company would take him to the crematorium for the committal. Some of the extended family were unhappy about this arrangement, but by letting them know the time and date they were able to connect with this ending by holding him in mind.

Until relatively recently, funerals were largely the domain of the Christian Church, and the minister would have been primarily responsible for making the necessary arrangements with the family. Now there is more choice about the kind of funeral someone wishes to have, and where the person has not been religious a non-religious or Humanist celebrant may take the service. It is not always straightforward for families to answer the question about whether or not they want a religious ceremony. There may be mixed views amongst the relatives, and between the family and the deceased.

Families only get one chance to do a funeral for a loved one, so it really matters to get it right. With so much choice and more of a market mentality in funeral taking, it can be even more confusing than ever for relatives. The father of a member of staff died. Her family had been offered a religious or non-religious ceremony by the funeral director, and they had felt some pressure to decide quickly. While the occasion had been acceptable, it seemed that it had not been entirely in keeping with what the family had hoped, and she was left with a degree of dissatisfaction about it. If the funeral is lacking, it is always possible to do something at a later date, a service of memorial or thanksgiving, or when the ashes are buried or scattered. Giving families this information can be very helpful.

I am sometimes surprised by the people who ask me to take a relative's funeral. A man in his early fifties was dying. He had told staff that he did not wish to see a chaplain when he was first admitted, and so I had of course respected his views. I met his mother and a friend sitting outside his room on one occasion. I was wearing a clerical shirt, as I always do, and we struck up a conversation. Tony's mother was clearly angry to be burying her son; it was the wrong way around. She said she couldn't believe in a God who could let this happen. I don't recall what I said, but I expect it was to show empathy with the difficult situation she was in. This was the only time we met, and the conversation lasted only a few minutes. I was astonished to be approached after Tony's death and asked to take his funeral. This suggests to me that it is the relationship that matters most to people, not the specifics of faith, doctrine or denomination. Somehow, in that brief conversation, I must have given the impression to Tony's mother that I would be able to respect the views of her son, whilst also offering her something meaningful.

The internet gives people access to all kinds of advice and guidance about organizing a funeral, from popular poems to suitable music.

Sometimes people think that if they want to choose non-biblical readings or non-religious music, this is incompatible with a Christian ceremony. I suspect that many perceive a religious funeral in terms of inaccessible language and long-winded sermons about the afterlife. Perhaps some clergy do take funerals like this, but I imagine many do not. Chaplain Tess Ward helpfully writes of three kinds of funeral: traditional religious (Christian), non-religious, led by a celebrant of no faith, and contemporary (Christian). The contemporary funeral includes the wishes of the family with regard to music, poems and eulogies but can have a religious element to it as well, some prayers, and a commendation and blessing.

I consider that a funeral must be pastorally appropriate and that whoever is in attendance must feel included in the ritual. At a funeral there are likely to be people with a wide range of views about faith, God and life after death. If I make a statement of Christian faith, I always acknowledge this diversity of views and may introduce my remarks by saying, "It is my belief, and perhaps yours . . . ". I hope that by doing so I am demonstrating a respect for difference, that having doubts or no faith is acceptable, and that I want everyone to feel included. So many people have issues with the Church, religion or God, that when they see me walking into the crematorium in clerical dress their hearts probably sink! Perhaps they are expecting lots of inaccessible God talk. The sooner I can disabuse them of that and make them feel comfortable and welcomed the better. I believe that the way a funeral is conducted, the compassion shown to the mourners and the respect shown to the deceased will demonstrate more clearly the love of God than using lots of words.

Funerals following a suicide

Taking a funeral after someone has died by suicide is always challenging. Given the history and attitude of the Christian Church towards suicide which I discussed in Chapter 4, families may feel more inclined to choose a non-religious celebrant. Whoever takes the service, and meets with the family to discuss it, will need to be skilled in pastoral listening, compassionate and without judgement.

Just as the pastor will be listening carefully to the family, so they too will be listening to you—to see if you believe there is any hope for their loved one. Can they be forgiven? Are they eternally damned? Do you blame the family for the suicide? The family will have many questions they would like to be able to ask the deceased, and many spiritual questions which they may want you to answer. This is not the time to dwell on doctrine, or to expound theological arguments, but to reach out with compassion and empathy into a heart-breaking situation, in the most loving way possible. What no one should do is to make this tragedy even worse. Acknowledging the enormity of everyone's pain, and showing solidarity in silence may be the only authentic pastoral response.

Given the feelings of shame that often accompany a suicide, the family may want the funeral to focus only on the person's life, and to gloss over the trauma of the death. While it is essential to respect the wishes of the family, it may also be important to acknowledge gently the pain of the situation for everyone—the deceased and those left behind—in the liturgy. There are some well-crafted collects, prayers and poems which can be helpful. Grieving relatives can be encouraged in the service to attend to and accept their emotions as they listen to music or keep silence. Sometimes symbolic actions like lighting a candle can be deeply meaningful.

The funeral after a suicide or any other traumatic death has particular functions. It allows the community to come together with the family, to offer support, solidarity and compassion. The service, and the one who leads it, somehow holds the shock and trauma, containing it and making it fractionally less overwhelming. The Christian liturgy points towards hope; for the deceased—with a loving, compassionate and understanding God, and for the family—that they will find a way through the darkness towards the light.

Funerals of the "unloved"

The preparations for a funeral I have described so far are for when there are people there to grieve, when the meaning of someone's life can be understood by the love they have given and received, attested to by the people present at the funeral. There have been and will always be funerals where there is no one to mourn. Perhaps because the person who has died has outlived all who knew them, perhaps because they have been estranged from everyone by choice or circumstance. In these cases what and who is the funeral for?

As a curate in East London, I was involved with the project for homeless people at our church. One of the regular clients to our day-centre died. Like many homeless men who have slept rough for many years, he had no contact with his family, even if they still existed. His project worker and I found out when his funeral was and decided to attend. His was to be a pauper's funeral, at the expense of the local council, so as minimalist as it could be. It was a pretty grey and overcast day, and the weather seemed to reflect the occasion. The funeral directors arrived with the body, which they were simply going to deliver to the crematorium for disposal. They were obviously surprised to see anyone there to acknowledge this man's death, and no minister had been tasked with committing his body into the hands of God. I was very new in position and had never taken a funeral before. I had rarely seen one taken, and I was not in the least prepared. However, my colleague and I felt that something needed to be said and done; we were incensed that he was otherwise being dismissed with no acknowledgement that his life had had any meaning. We persuaded the funeral directors to let me say something. I've no idea what I did in the end, but that barely mattered, what did matter was that we were there with the intention to respect his life and his death and commit him to God's compassionate keeping. What happened that day made no difference to the deceased, but it made a difference to me and, I suspect, my colleague. No matter what the circumstances of this man's life, or the loneliness of his death on the streets of London, he was and always will be a child of God and deserved the same respect as if there were hundreds at his funeral.

This experience and the strength of feelings it stirred in me then, and continues to generate in me now, all these years later, probably impacted on the way I took funerals for prisoners when I came to HMP Isle of Wight, where prisoners were virtually all sex offenders. I commend the prison service for the way it deals with the funeral of a prisoner. Generally, unless the family wish otherwise, the prison will pay for the funeral. It will be a basic funeral, but if there are relatives who wish for more, the family must pay the difference. Sometimes prisoners would be returned to their home areas, and the funeral conducted by a local minister, so support for the family could continue afterwards. Some of the prisoners had no family who wanted to take any ownership of the funeral, or even attend. The nature of their offences or the concern about media attention, and additional shame for the families, meant that funerals could take place quietly, away from scrutiny, on the Isle of Wight. This meant that often I was taking a funeral where I had no contact with any family member, and the only information I could gather about the person was from their fellow prisoners or staff at the prison.

Generally, I was accompanied to a funeral by a senior member of staff from the prison, and due respect was paid to the person, regardless of their offence. I said prayers and a few words, acknowledging that God is merciful and gracious, and understands the secrets of our hearts and lives, better than we like to admit. I am not there to pass judgement on anyone, in life or in death. I am there to commend them to God's care and keeping and to leave the rest to God. There have been occasions where the prisoner has requested that no ceremony is conducted. I have still been present on these occasions, just to stand as the coffin is brought in and the curtains are drawn, and to say a prayer to myself in silence feels important. Even if the prisoner has felt that his life had no meaning or done nothing worthy of positive comment, God knows and cares.

I took the funeral of a prisoner who was a prolific paedophile. No one came to his funeral except his brother, out of a sense of duty perhaps, or a desire to see him disposed of? Some would say I was burying a monster, and there is no doubt that his actions had been monstrous, and he had harmed scores of people. Was there anything positive to say about the man? I also took his memorial service in the prison. Prisoners could not leave the prison to attend one another's funerals, of course, so we always held a memorial gathering for them in the prison afterwards. I always invited those attending to share their thoughts or memories of the person. At the memorial for this prisoner, his contemporaries described him as generous, respectful and helpful to others on the wing. I sometimes wished that the families who had been so ashamed of their relatives could hear from others that their relative had done some good to others; perhaps it might have brought them some comfort?

Other kinds of rituals

There are many kinds of ritual and occasions for them. Norman, an atheist, asked to see me. He had many issues with religion that he wanted to unpack in his remaining days. In the course of our conversations, he disclosed to me people in his past who had caused him harm and of whom he found it hard let go. He requested that we visit the chapel in the hospice and that I should create a ritual to acknowledge that he had forgiven them. This ritual was not to include any God language, and could not involve the lighting of candles, as he was having to use an oxygen cylinder to breathe.

Anointing someone who is dying, with oil, and making the sign of the cross on their head or hands, can be a way of blessing the patient and a symbolic gesture of letting go. It may reconnect the patient, or their loved ones, with a faith in God and remind them of the greater presence of love who is with them always. Words of commendation of the patient into the arms of a loving God can bring comfort and reassurance and may ease the sense of panic in either the patient or the people they are leaving behind. It is a symbol of hope in the face of despair, and a pointer to peace amidst the chaos and confusion of parting.

Duncan was very agitated. He had been so fearful of losing control in his final days that he had tried to end his own life rather than wait for death to come naturally. He did not succeed and came to the hospice. Duncan and his wife had a Christian faith, and she asked me to come and visit him. I asked her if she would like me to say some prayers and anoint him. I used traditional words to accompany the anointing, which included acknowledgement of sins, and the absolution of forgiveness. I hummed a familiar tune and sang a hymn that he knew; I read Psalm 23, and we said the Lord's Prayer. Duncan had been unresponsive, though agitated for several days, and as I prayed he opened his eyes, held my gaze for a few moments, and said "Amen". The contrast in Duncan's state before and after this ritual was astonishing. He slept peacefully afterwards for four hours, something he had not done for days, and died shortly afterwards.

In the Anglican tradition, on Maundy Thursday the clergy and lay leaders of the Church gather in their local cathedral to renew the vows of their vocation and to receive blessed oils which will then be used for anointing the sick and dying throughout the year. I may explain this to families in the hospice as I anoint their relative, and it reminds them that they, and their loved one, are connected to a wider community of faith, of which they are a part. It is not always possible to anoint a patient before they die, and there have been occasions when a family have requested prayers for their relative shortly after their death, either in the room of the hospice or in the chapel of rest. This may or may not take place with the family present.

In a pluralist society with people who may have no faith or for whom the language of God is unfamiliar or unacceptable, there may still be a need, often not expressed, for ritual. I was asked by someone without a faith to conduct a ritual at the end of life; they felt it was necessary for their loved one to help them let go, and for themselves as they sought to release them. In this instance, I have used poetry or music or a phrase that has meaning, such as "we let you go" repeated in rhythm or response. This may be more helpful and profound than repeating the Lord's Prayer or Psalm 23. Sometimes I sense the actual words used are of less significance at that intense moment, than the way they are said and the manner in which that situation is conducted.

Rituals of remembering

Funerals are not the only rituals of remembering. At times of national or international tragedy, some people may feel the need to gather to do something. It may be to light candles in a public place, or a place of worship; to place flowers or soft toys at a site of a disaster or by the road when there has been a fatal accident. The ritual of remembering matters, not only to those immediately involved but to the community, however that is defined.

Grief and loss are very isolating experiences, and people can feel lonely and at odds with the rest of the world around them. Rituals which enable people who have been through a similar loss to come together and remember can help to reduce those feelings for a while. In our hospice we have memorial services every quarter for people whose relatives have died in recent months and annual events for remembering. Symbolic actions like lighting candles or placing thoughts of loved ones on a tree can help to remind someone who is grieving that the one lost is not forgotten. Anniversaries of death, or significant dates associated with the deceased, are painful, and often bereaved people don't know what to do on these occasions. Should they stay indoors and shut themselves in with their sorrow? Should they go to a place that has significance and weep or remember? Should they seek out people and experiences that will distract them? Should they go to the burial ground and talk to their beloved? There is no right answer, and each person has to find their own way through those difficult days. If something gets them through then it may become a tradition, a habit that they repeat.

In prison people who are grieving have very few options available to them on an anniversary. They cannot stay in their cells if they are in a working prison, there are no family members with them to remember and reminisce together. They might be able to speak to a relative on the phone, and if they are fortunate someone might book a visit near the day. Then they will be in a public hall, full of people, where showing emotion, even offering a comforting touch may not be possible. Often prisoners will ask a chaplain to take them to the chapel on a significant date, to light a candle and spend a few minutes in prayer or silent reflection. They might want to talk about the person, share stories of their life, or express their regrets about the relationship. Prisoners often find it hard to trust other people, to show vulnerability in front of others and to express emotion openly. A chaplain may be one of the very few people that they will open up to, and on an occasion such as this it may be very important for them to do so.

I was asked to take a young woman to the chapel in Holloway. Rachel had had a miscarriage. At around the date when the child would have been born, she asked to come to the chapel and light a candle. She was not only sad at the loss of her baby, she was filled with guilt because she felt that her chaotic life and drug taking had caused the child's death. Lighting a candle fulfilled her need to acknowledge her grief, but she also wanted to confess what she felt was her part in the child's death and she needed to hear words of forgiveness. The sadness at her loss was more poignant than ever for me, as I myself was visibly pregnant at the time. Rachel was one of many women who used drugs or alcohol, who after detoxing became more in tune with the pains of losses they had experienced, which their addictions had previously suppressed or masked. In this ritual, hopefully, Rachel was able to acknowledge her past, believe herself forgiven, forgive herself, and move on with the rest of her life.

Theological reflection

After Jesus' death the women in his party of followers intend to anoint his body with oils, a gesture of love and kindness, and to show respect for his body as is customary in the Jewish tradition. This would have been acceptable and expected as part of the rituals of mourning.

The anointing of the body before being wrapped in a linen shroud and laid in the tomb is a process called *tohorah*. The oils and aromatic herbs would have helped to stave off the rapid process of bodily decomposition associated with being in a hot climate.

In Mark's Gospel, when Jesus is in the house of Simon the Leper, a woman anoints Jesus' head with a costly ointment which she has brought in an alabaster jar. This ritual is shocking to those present. It is an audacious act, considered wasteful and reckless. A woman has broken into a male domain, and the onlookers are angry. But Jesus speaks in her defence, and says that she has performed a good service to him. "She has done what she could; she has anointed my body beforehand for its burial." (Mark 14:8). Jesus links the actions of the woman with the ritual of *tohorah*. This must have further shocked the guests at the party. This ritual was associated with death, and not with the living.

Like a sacrament in the Christian tradition, rituals can be outward signs of inner change. Jesus had to explain the ritual to the guests at the party. He found deep significance in her actions – they mirrored those of the women who would anoint his body after his death. Just as this ritual prepares Jesus for his death, so he uses the meaning of this act to prepare his followers who witness it, for the reality of what is to come.

In end-of-life rituals that I have conducted in the hospice, there is this same symbolic preparation; sometimes it is for the patient, to enable them to have some peace or acceptance of their situation; sometimes it is to prepare the onlookers for the fact that death is approaching. Those who are close to death can rarely articulate what these rituals do for them. However, dying is an art and not a science and predicting the moment when death is closest, and it is the right time to perform these rituals, is not straightforward.

Rosa seemed to be dying, so I said prayers and anointed her, as the family requested. She seemed unresponsive, but when I had finished she opened her eyes and said, "That was lovely." She recovered sufficiently afterwards to spend a happy week at home with her family, and when she returned to the hospice, on two further occasions I said similar prayers with her. Fortunately, the family were very good-natured about this, and we were able to laugh at the situation subsequently.

What actually transpires in those deeply personal and intimate moments of ritual can barely be described. It is often a moment of holiness which perhaps can only be understood by God. In the same way, the woman who anointed Jesus may not have been conscious of the meaning of her act, but she recognized it as significant, something she felt compelled to do for one she loved.

Someone who accompanies a dying person, and the dying person themselves, is standing in a liminal place; a threshold between what is known and what is unknown. It is a place of uncertainty and waiting, a place of discomfort, but also of potential and transformation. Many people find it hard to inhabit this space. Many don't know what to say, or do, or how to be. As a priest or pastor, it is a domain in which and with which we need to be comfortable. We don't have tasks to perform, or medication to administer like the doctors, nurses and healthcare assistants, but we do bring an authority from having been in this space before. Sometimes just chatting and being visibly accepting of whatever is happening can be helpful. We can also offer rituals such as anointing, laying on hands, and prayers, which can help those who are less familiar and at ease with liminality to feel more peaceful and accepting of the mystery that is death itself and what, if anything, lies beyond.

CHAPTER 8

Caring for Yourself as a Pastoral Carer

In this chapter I draw from my own experience of more than twenty years in ministry to discuss the importance emotionally, psychologically, spiritually and theologically of self-care and self-compassion. I share some of the things that have helped me to remain resilient, and I describe the essential components of care for pastoral carers.

Self-care

As a chaplain or a pastor who is caring for others it is vital to look after yourself; failure to do so can easily lead to burnout. Many of us put up barriers to doing things to look after ourselves: we are too busy; we feel guilty if we do; we take rather too literally the command to be the servant of all. My particular challenge has been the guilt of being a full-time working mother and absent from the home for long periods. So perhaps my "hobbies", especially when the children were very young, were putting them to bed, reading bedtime stories and playing. As the children are now older and have found their own interests I need to discover activities for myself; writing being one such interest.

As well as practical self-care and good time management, there is also internal self-care: developing self-awareness; skills of reflection; maintaining emotional boundaries. People sometimes wonder how I or others manage to work full-time in environments whose sole purpose is to care for the dying or with people in prison. Perhaps the key requirement is resilience, which is defined as the ability to recover quickly from difficulties. In a challenging environment, such as a prison, where I started my chaplaincy ministry, this is an essential skill to acquire, otherwise one would easily be overwhelmed. In HMP Holloway, a busy local women's prison, you could move from one emotionally challenging conversation to the next in relentless succession. Building up resilience happens almost imperceptibly. I learned to make the most of the travelling time between walking from one wing to the next, or in the hospice I might make a detour back from the inpatient unit to the chapel for a few minutes before returning to the ward to see another patient. The geography of the hospice is more conducive to this sort of approach than a prison where a detour may take you half an hour out of your way, with numerous doors and gates to unlock en route!

Developing emotional boundaries is crucial for your own well-being when dealing with anyone in distress, whether or not they are dying. It can be tempting when listening to someone else's story to see yourself in their situation so completely that instead of listening to the other person your thoughts and imagination take over, and before you realize you are thinking about how you would cope in their position. This is when you are not only dealing with the distress of someone else, you are dealing with your own imagined pain and that becomes overwhelming. I find this happens more when the person I am with is like me, or like someone important to me. There was an elderly man who was dying in the hospice. I'd seen him a few times and found myself feeling more sad and emotional with him than with some other patients. I realized on reflection that he reminded me of my father. Once I identified this response, I was more able to understand my reaction.

Listening is hard work, and there are times when my mind drifts away from what the person is telling me. It can be hard to pull yourself back from getting sidetracked by your own thoughts. It is preferable to prevent yourself from being distracted in the first place. Recognizing why I am reacting in a particular way can be helpful: am I drifting off because I am tired? Is the venue making me sleepy? Can I open the window? Do I need to eat something? Am I bored? If so, why?

I have learned to understand the language of transference, projection and self-awareness, not from academic study or training particularly but by working alongside others who are trained in this terminology both as colleagues and as mentors. In Chapter 2, I use eight terms which are essential elements in establishing a therapeutic relationship with another person. I want to now use these same terms in caring for ourselves.

Attentiveness

Being attentive to another requires me to listen to my own thoughts and to recognize my own reactions: physical, emotional and spiritual. Sometimes people will say things about their lives or actions that make me feel tearful, even when the other person is dry-eyed, and then I need to be aware of whether the sadness is in me or is a projection from the person I am listening to. Having wise guides and counsellors who will help me to attend to my own reactions, to ask me why some person or situation has affected or impacted on me in a particular way, can really help me to develop this deep self-awareness.

In theological terms it is important to ask what God is saying to me in this situation. I have found that using the Ignatian spiritual exercise of examen is a valuable tool for paying attention to God. In this exercise you ask yourself what you are most grateful for, or what has given you most life today. And then you consider what you are least grateful for, or what has not been life-affirming. Paying attention to both responses, especially encouraging myself to reflect on the less comfortable position of the things that have disturbed me, has been an invaluable way of paying attention to God.

Active listening

I recognize how important it is for me to be listened to at depth myself. I need someone else to listen, concentrate and understand what I am talking about and to be as observant of my needs as I am of others'. It is not right or appropriate to hear other people's stories of distress, without having somewhere that I can take this to offload and to think about. I need to be heard in order to listen.

Accompaniment

I need to be accompanied, by others and by God, in order to be alongside those to whom I minister. Using this term in a musical sense, an accompaniment gives body and wholeness to a solo instrument to enrich and broaden the sound. If I play unaccompanied, then I am more likely to get out of tune or to alter the tempo. I find this a helpful metaphor for thinking about care for the one who cares. If I reflect on those who have accompanied me as soul-friends and work supervisors, I can see how they have provided the background to my ministry and have enriched the care that I have been able to offer to others.

Authenticity

When I am being listened to, I need to be able to be completely myself, without the expectations or projections people place on me as a priest and chaplain. I must be able to be honest, free to say whatever I need to say at that particular moment, using whatever language I need to without feeling judged. I need to be able to go somewhere to bawl my eyes out at a situation that has made me very sad, or to swear at length at a situation that has enraged me. I need a "no holds barred" space and place to let out a week, a year or a decade's worth of emotions. I also need the person who is listening to me to be authentic.

Compassion

Having self-compassion is as vital to ministry as having compassion for others. I have to learn to accept myself, warts and all, if I am going to accept, and indeed love, others with faults similar to my own. It is not just a cosy statement of Jesus' to "love your neighbour as yourself" (Matthew 22.39). It is a common-sense approach to genuinely caring. If I cannot love myself; if I cannot accept the parts of me which I find difficult to acknowledge, then how can I honestly love someone else? Richard Rohr put it succinctly:

> Trying to love others without a foundational reverence for yourself ends up as neediness, manipulation, and unsustainable infatuation, expressing itself in endless battles of co-dependency. Trying to love yourself and not to love others is what we mean by narcissism.[8]

Self-compassion allows me to make mistakes and to learn from them! It helps me to listen to the advice which I readily give out to others. Self-compassion helps me to recognize when I am getting over-tired and irritable. Self-compassion prompts me to take annual leave, to meet up with friends or go for a walk, without feeling guilty. Self-compassion is a life-saving technique to develop. It is not self-indulgence or self-pity. It is realizing that I am not indispensable, that I don't need to work for twice as many hours as anyone else in order to justify my existence. I don't need to be on call every day, 365 days a year, and reading work emails whilst on holiday. These are the ego dangers of ministry and care which must be challenged at all costs in others, and probably most importantly in myself.

Containment

If I am to be able to contain the emotions of others, many others, then I need to have spaces where my own feelings can be held safely. When caring for others I can feel like a sponge soaking up their pains and sadness, and I need places to wring myself out emotionally before I can absorb anything else. If I don't do this, then I will become saturated with feelings, often projected ones, and be of no use to myself or anyone around me, loved ones included. Containment is providing me with the opportunity to let go and leave behind strong feelings. It is so important for me to know what this feels like personally, so that I can understand what it feels like for those that I care for. I need the person who is listening to me to be self-confident and assured about themselves, so that I don't have to worry about them. If I have concerns about them, then I will slip into the role of being a pastoral listener, and I will not be able to get what I need in that encounter. Feeling contained means feeling safe, and as I am listened to I need to know that what I say will not be repeated outside of the room.

Challenge

Everyone in ministry needs people who will challenge them in order to keep them grounded and humble. I have needed people to ask me difficult questions about what I am doing and why. I have needed people to challenge me to have more self-compassion, to recognize in myself the signs of burning out or to consider whether I need to move on from a particular work situation. I have needed my husband to challenge me to invest in our relationship and my children to challenge me to pay them more attention. I have accepted these challenges, because they have come from people who love me and care for me. If I had not been challenged by others, I would probably not have lasted this long in this kind of intense ministry.

Companionship

In addition to the seven elements I highlight in Chapter 2 for establishing a pastoral relationship, when caring for oneself companionship is an essential addition. Some kinds of ministry can be very isolating and lonely. Finding the right people to share the load of responsibility can be very supportive, and recognizing that others have a part to play in caring can help to maintain a sense of perspective. In our spiritual care team meetings in the hospice, we provide space for reflection on the work we do and the situations we face. One person might share with the team a pastoral situation with which they are beginning to feel overwhelmed; as we listen to each other we begin to see that others have also been involved in the support of this individual too and the perspective changes. It can be a timely reminder to us that we each contribute to the spiritual care of the patients and their families, as do many others in the multi-disciplinary team, and that no one person carries all the weight of support. When we recognize this, we avoid the pitfall of feeling indispensable, we feel more able to share the load, and it keeps us grounded and humble.

Types of support

Everyone will discover their own support needs. Lots of people will only learn that they need to care for themselves after they have become burned out, or lost faith in themselves or in God. In the next section I will share some of the ways in which I have received support throughout my ministry. I know that I will continue to need this care if I am to remain in this kind of work. If there are other people in ministry who are doing similar work and who have none of the five support strategies described below then I would be asking serious questions about their ability to do the work to the best of their ability; I would question the quality of the work that they do, and I would be concerned for their emotional, psychological and spiritual wellbeing.

Work supervision

Work supervision is not the same as managerial supervision in the workplace and should not be confused with it. It is not something that should be picked up when necessary. It is necessary for it to be there all the time, at regular intervals. I would ideally have monthly supervision for an hour as a minimum.

In work supervision the supervisor needs to be trustworthy and competent; non-judgemental but challenging; separate from the organization in which I am working, but have an understanding of it. They need to maintain confidentiality and to have sympathy for my theological standpoint, even if it is not shared.

For a short period, I received supervision from a colleague working in the same hospice. After a few months we both recognized that the situation should not continue; there might be patients that we both supported, or groups we worked together on, which meant that the boundaries were blurred. We needed to be able to relate as colleagues for these matters, and the supervisory role confused this relationship. I looked for supervision outside the organization which was more appropriate and safer.

In my own ministry, work supervision is something I have always sought for myself; it is only in the hospice that it has been actively encouraged. I found a supervisor while I was a curate and have maintained that pattern throughout my ministry. When I moved to a new area into a different kind of chaplaincy, in a university, and could not find a work supervisor, I felt far less supported emotionally and spiritually; this was not healthy for those with whom I was working or for myself. Work supervision may have a cost implication, since many work environments will not pay for it, though they may allow time to attend it. I believe that it is money well spent, and rather than questioning the financial cost of having to pay for it, I would question the emotional cost of not having it at all. In my own case, work supervision has been my most valuable tool for self-development, self-awareness, self-reflection; it is probably the single most important thing that has kept me going in this kind of ministry. Work supervision is not mandatory for chaplains. I think it should be.

Spiritual direction

Spiritual direction is as important to me as work supervision. It is sometimes referred to as having a soul-friend, or soul midwifery. In spiritual direction it is essential that there is a shared faith perspective. It is a space where I am encouraged to reflect theologically as well as emotionally, and it is in this relationship where I try to discern my vocation and life-choices. Here I will be challenged about my prayer life, encouraged to nourish my spirituality and reminded to take regular retreats. Here I am asked to think about my understanding of God and to listen to what God is asking of me. It is also a place where I can be held and heard. In these conversations, there is theological depth and spiritual challenge. For me the importance of a spiritual director is that they know me well. I know some people have spiritual directors for decades. I first met my current spiritual director when I was training to be ordained and went to his church on placement. He has seen me grow into ministry and has supported my development, the highs and spiritual lows, with loving-kindness. I try to see my spiritual director three or four times a year. Knowing that he is praying for me throughout the year is wonderfully supportive.

Counselling

I have also had counselling at various times in my life. Initially, I started in my early twenties, and then I struggled to accept that I needed it. It helped me to discern a direction for my life as well as supporting me during a period of depression. I look back at this experience as a formative time of self-development. I now see any talking therapy as helpful and those who seek it out can be doing so from the strength of self-awareness and self-care, not from an inability to deal with life or a sign of weakness. My own positive experiences of counselling have given me confidence to suggest it to many others who have come to talk to me. I would also consider having counselling again, if I recognized a need in myself to do so, or if others in my supportive circle thought I needed this kind of additional support.

Retreats

Those of us who are in full-time ministry in the Church are generally encouraged to take an annual retreat. I have been very bad about doing this myself. It was only when I felt completely stuck in a situation, and on the verge of slipping back into a depression, that I took the positive step of going on a retreat. Diving in at the deep end, I went to St Beuno's Jesuit Spirituality Centre in North Wales for a ten-day silent guided Ignatian retreat. The only time I spoke during those ten days was for forty-five minutes each day with a spiritual guide. It was a life-changing experience and helped me to listen to God at great depth and in doing so to discern a way forward in my situation. In the same way that everyone will find their own way of praying, so not everyone will feel drawn to Ignatian spirituality, but for me it was a "coming home" and a momentous movement from a head-led understanding of faith to a heart-experienced encounter with God.

If my experience at St Beuno's is anything to go by, such retreats are to be handled with care, for this was no easy ride of self-indulgence; it was painfully hard work, intensely exhausting at times, but ultimately liberating and life-affirming. There were moments when I felt that I couldn't go on, and I felt so unwell that I thought I should go home, but I stayed and eventually found peace and renewed strength. It was an experience like the "dark night of the soul" which St John of the Cross sought to describe. I see now that I could not have made the move into hospice chaplaincy without going through this experience: to move on from a situation that was life-destroying, to have courage to step out into the unknown and trust God completely.

Cell group

When I was at theological college, we were encouraged to form "cell groups". These were small groups of ordinands who would meet regularly to reflect theologically together. I have been in the same group for more than twenty years, and although some participants have come and gone, there are three of the original group remaining. We now meet once a year for forty-eight hours to share our journeys together. We have watched one another's relationships blossom, lives develop and parents die. We have supported one another through many changes of job and home, and it has been a unique and invaluable part of the journey through ordained ministry.

We developed a pattern of listening when we first started meeting, where we gave each other a set amount of time to speak without interruption, and then the group would offer comment or reflection on what each has said. We pray together and share Communion together. We eat together and go for a walk together. We may have little contact with one another in between our gatherings, but knowing that we are there for each other, has been a great blessing.

Theological reflection

There is a body of theology which emphasizes the self-emptying and service of ministry and the Christian life. Taken to extremes this can encourage a carer to become a martyr, or to seek emotional or spiritual affirmation from others or from God by being heroic. People who might advocate this approach of self-denial may look to the actions of Jesus' ministry as example and justification. I want to look at the stories of Jesus' ministry to consider a different approach.

From the beginning of his public ministry Jesus chose people to accompany him. Often the disciples are seen as an inner circle of followers, ones who had the opportunity to have greater insight into who Jesus really was, and who would aid the mission of the gospel; they were the ones who would become fishers of people. In John's Gospel, however, and particularly in the final discourses in John 13–17 there is a tenderness and intimacy in tone in which we see the followers of Jesus as not simply agents of spreading the good news, but as close friends of Jesus himself.

> I do not call you servants any longer, because the servant does not know what the master is doing; but I have called you friends, because I have made known to you everything that I have heard from my Father.
>
> *John 15:15*

Jesus needed people around him for companionship, love and support. It was certainly Jesus' faith in God that sustained him, but the humanity of Jesus meant that he needed the accompaniment of people who knew and understood him better than most. Jesus had much to teach and share, but he also needed receptive people to listen. His friends did not always say or do the right thing, but they did remind Jesus to take care of himself, and helped to provide for his own physical and emotional needs.

In the house at Bethany, home to Mary, Martha and Lazarus, we see clearly Jesus' relationships of depth with his friends. Among these people there are the most intimate of stories, and in this place we see Jesus most fully at home. This house is mentioned frequently in the Gospels, a home that was quite unusual for being a place where women's voices and presence are given prominence. This is the home where Mary listened and Martha cared. Both were necessary for Jesus; Martha looked after him physically, Mary absorbed his message (Luke 10:38–41). Martha was not overawed by the charisma of Jesus; she challenged him, both on this occasion where she sought his support to get her sister to help in the kitchen, and later when she scolded him for not coming to see them sooner when her brother was ill (John 11:21). It was in seeing the impact of the death of Lazarus and the sorrow of his sister's grief that Jesus is most vulnerable himself.

> When Jesus saw her weeping, and the Jews who came with her also weeping, he was greatly disturbed in spirit and deeply moved.
> *John 11:33*

It was in this home, after Lazarus had been raised from the dead, that Mary anointed Jesus with costly ointment, and wiped his feet with her hair (John 12:3). It is among this family that we sense Jesus' needs for friendship, companionship, warmth of human love and intimacy being met, and it was also in the context of this very human setting that his divinity was revealed and he was glorified (John 11:4).

Jesus' whole ministry was developed through sharing human relationships. He never conducted his ministry in isolation. He did not preciously guard the teaching and ministry for himself, he included and involved others, recognizing and affirming their capability to spread the gospel and share the load. When Jesus sent the twelve disciples out to preach and to heal, he sent them out in twos, acknowledging that each of us needs support when asked to carry out demanding missions.

When they returned Jesus showed sensitive compassion for their care and recuperation. He recognized the need for a balanced approach to ministry, and for the need to withdraw and be, rather than to be always active and doing.

> The apostles gathered around Jesus, and told him all that they had done and taught. He said to them, "Come away to a deserted place all by yourselves and rest a while." For many were coming and going, and they had no leisure even to eat.
>
> *Mark 6:30, 31*

Jesus also knew his own need for solitude and silence, and for time to be away from the crowds, and even from his closest friends. After the feeding of the crowd we are told that Jesus "made his disciples get into the boat and go ahead to the other side, to Bethsaida, while he dismissed the crowd. After saying farewell to them, he went up the mountain to pray" (Mark 6:45,46).

At the start of his ministry, in the wilderness, and at the end of his active ministry in the Garden of Gethsemane, we see Jesus wrestling with inner struggles of conviction and faith—facing his deepest torments and anguish of heart. These testing experiences happen when Jesus withdraws to a lonely place, and when he himself experiences the dark night of the soul. From these experiences he finds the courage and faith to begin his ministry, and to face his mortality.

Jesus models for us not only self-giving and self-emptying, but self-care, in his need for friendship, loyal and honest support, companionship and challenge. He also demonstrates the need for solitude and space with God. We are not called to be superheroes and we are certainly not invincible. Those who care most effectively for others are probably those who are most aware of their own fragility, vulnerability and humanity. This is the concept of "the wounded healer", which Henri Nouwen writes about. We are asked to trust in God, not to play at being God. As pastoral carers, it is as important, for each of us, to follow Jesus' example and to have balance in our lives, and perspective on ourselves, in our care for others.

CHAPTER 9

Facing Taboos

A taboo is a word or action that is avoided for social or religious reasons. In this book, as I have reflected on pastoral care, I have been confronting the taboo subjects of prison and death. In this chapter I want to consider why these subjects are still taboo, and why it is important to us as a society and as individuals to talk more about them. I also discuss the roles and perceptions of hospices and prisons for society and reflect theologically about the meaning of taboos in the Gospels.

Death as a taboo subject

All history, literature, philosophy and religion, as well as medical science, reminds us of this one truth: that the death of the body is an inevitability. Yet somehow most of us choose to forget it, so that when death looms closer, it always come as a shock, and we feel cheated by its arrival—too soon.

The modern hospice movement, which has been in existence for more than fifty years, has recognized that when people have thought about death and prepared themselves and their families for it, they will face this inevitability with greater equanimity, and the pain of grief for their relatives may be eased. Hospices have sought to encourage greater openness and confidence in talking about death; so why is it that in 2019 doctors are found to be poorly equipped to talk to their patients about death and need to be encouraged to bring up the subject of dying earlier in a patient's treatment?[9] And why do the relatives of an elderly frail woman who has recently had a stroke tell her that she is being morbid if she wants to talk about her funeral arrangements? Why do we try to disguise the existence of death by using euphemisms like "passing" instead of the word itself? As well as the hospice movement, there have been initiatives in recent years such as the Dying Matters campaign and Death Cafés, each seeking to encourage people to talk about and prepare for death. Have they made any significant inroads into changing attitudes towards death or making it less taboo?

In many cultures, death is a more present reality, with people having shorter life expectancies due to poverty, hunger and poor living conditions. Perhaps people living in these situations have more experience of death so integrate it more into their understanding of life? Perhaps our modern, affluent, scientifically advanced society creates the illusion that we are invincible and masks the reality of death or makes it seem more remote? The language that people use around illness is often that of conflict: I am going to fight this cancer; this condition is not going to beat me. This defiance in the face of an illness, whilst arguably encouraging the person to remain positive, also hides the fact that although they may win this particular battle, they certainly will not win the war!

Hospice as a taboo place

Cicely Saunders saw the need to provide good care to people at the end of their lives, to treat them holistically and to enable them to die as pain-free and peacefully as possible. To those that require and use the services of a hospice, either in their own home, or in the hospice itself, this kind of care is generally warmly welcomed and well-received. However, until people have need of the hospice, or have to visit others there, many are fearful of entering its doors, and some even refuse to do so. This may be because they believe that the hospice is a place of distress or because they see the hospice itself as a taboo.

Prison as a taboo place

The conversation topic of prisons is not a taboo in itself, but it is one that generates strong feelings in people. Everyone has an opinion about prisons, what they are there to do; who is or should be in them; whether or not they should be more punitive. Most people have an impression of what they are like, though they may never have been inside one; and they use strong language about the kind of people that are held there.

Prisons contain people who have been accused of committing or who have committed crimes. Many of these crimes are societal and religious taboos: rape; murder; violence; abuse. These are subjects that, like death, people don't want to talk about, or if they do, it will be in strongly-worded language to distance themselves from the perpetrators. Labelling people as "monsters", "paedos" or "nonces" helps to separate those who are considered to be evil from the good in a dualistic way. It helps us to keep our distance from others—divides people into us and them, and perpetuates the myth that they are nothing like me.

The fact that people who have committed terrible offences are locked away means that as a society and individuals we feel safer. The fact that most of these same people will one day be released may be forgotten. According to Her Majesty's Prison Service, the primary purpose of a prison is to keep those sentenced to prison in custody—to protect the public—and to help prisoners lead law-abiding and useful lives, both while they are in prison and after they are released. This suggests that prisons exist to enable change, reformation and even healing. However, there are many in society and in politics who argue that people are sent to prison to be punished—and they believe that if this were to be reflected more in the regime, prison would become more of a deterrent.

In my life and ministry, I seem to have been drawn towards people and institutions that deal with societal taboos. I worked with people with HIV and AIDS when I was training for ordination, with people who were homeless in my curacy and then as chaplain in prisons and a hospice. I have had to confront and think about subjects and situations that most people would choose to avoid. It has been my way of educating myself and challenging my own prejudices. By meeting people who are dealing with life's taboos themselves in their lived experiences, I have seen beyond the labels and heard their human stories. Recognizing someone else's humanity, and acknowledging the similarities to myself rather than the differences between us, is the best antidote to dualistic—us and them—thinking that I have yet discovered.

Prisons and hospices in society

The outside of a prison looks imposing, with high walls and barbed wire on the top of them. You cannot look behind the walls of a prison unless you are a prisoner or a member of staff. A hospice, on the other hand, does everything to invite people in; the doors are always open; the activities are for everyone; the environment is welcoming. The prison exists to keep the public safe by keeping the people held within it inside. The greatest damage to a prison's reputation is when a prisoner escapes, as this will impact on the public confidence in the prison's security. The hospice needs the local community to value its work and to support it financially. Any reputational damage, such as if someone was not well cared for or not treated fairly, might impact on the public perception, and the hospice's ability to raise funds and continue providing the same quality of end-of-life care.

It is interesting to notice the public response to both kinds of establishments. Having worked on the Isle of Wight in both prison and hospice, I am in a unique position perhaps to observe these differences. There used to be three separate prisons on the Isle of Wight: Camp Hill, Parkhurst and Albany. They are located in the same area of the island, with only a few hundred metres between each of them, but they had entirely different atmospheres, types of prisoners and levels of security. Until 2009, when they became one prison managerially, they were run separately and might as well have been hundreds of miles apart. The vast majority of prisoners housed in these prisons came from the mainland. For a small community with a population of 140,000 to have three prisons must be quite unusual, if not unique. Many people living on the island were employed in the prisons or must have known someone who was.

Mountbatten Hospice, or the Earl Mountbatten Hospice as it was formerly known, has only been in existence on the Isle of Wight since

1982. Despite the taboo of the hospice itself and the taboos of death which it deals with, there is great pride and interest in the hospice amongst the island population. The number of people involved in volunteering for the organization, or who fund-raise for it, is incredible. Most island residents will have had some contact with the hospice, by knowing someone who has been supported by it, or by knowing someone who volunteers or works there. As a local charity it has a high profile, and in the local press there are frequently stories or pictures of people who have contributed in some way to the organization. It is a charity which is somehow "owned" by the community. The staff and the volunteers who work in the hospice are given discounts in shops and on ferries, and the logo of the hospice is proudly displayed in many locations. The words people use to describe the hospice are "like a five-star hotel", or even "heaven", the care provided is exemplary, and the nurses are often described as "angels". The hospice is light and airy, and people who come here for the first time are surprised that it is such an attractive and welcoming place. One visitor to the hospice said that before she came she thought it would be like a workhouse, with dark corridors where dead people were wheeled around on their way to the mortuary!

Staff who work in the prison are often reluctant to talk about their work, even where they work, to other people. Sometimes this is for security reasons, but largely it is because to disclose this in a pub or social gathering could lead to conversations about the work that staff do not wish to engage in, or which they cannot talk about for reasons of confidentiality. The public may not understand why someone works in the prison, and given that the majority of prisoners at HMP Isle of Wight are now sex offenders, they may be even less comprehending. People may question staff saying, "Why do you want to work there with that lot?" Staff have to deal with their own feelings about the offences of the prisoners, and at times this can be difficult; having to explain this to people who have little understanding or empathy towards them can be very hard. The public perception of a prison officer would probably be a tough male jailer, possibly an ex-serviceman, or perhaps a character from the TV programme of the 1970s, *Porridge*. Although prison officers are public servants, they are not regarded in the same way as fire-fighters or police, who have a more prominent and obvious role in protecting the public; perhaps because prisons and prison officers are out of sight, they are out of the public mind.

People in the community are much more sympathetic towards people who work in the hospice. They find it hard to imagine how people, particularly the nurses, can work continuously amongst people who are dying. The public image of a hospice nurse would be female, friendly, gentle, kind, compassionate and selfless. The role of a hospice nurse is regarded as a caring profession, even a vocation, in a way that can idealize those who work there. People may well look at the nursing staff as worthy of praise and affirmation, in a way that would rarely be the case for prison staff.

Reporting about the prison in the local paper is much less frequent than reporting about the hospice; generally, it is when there are significant negative events such as a concerted indiscipline, a higher number of assaults on prison staff, or when there are issues of overcrowding. How anything is reported about a prison is highly contentious; often decisions made within the context of a prison are measured by how it would be perceived in the public domain. When something positive happens in the prison, such as a community event, like a concert for the prisoners, there is a great deal of anxiety about whether or not the public would regard this as a waste of taxpayers' money. Would the negative responses from the public towards such an occasion outweigh the value to the prisoners' rehabilitation? Often the public will argue that law-abiding pensioners or hard-working people on low incomes do not have the same opportunities as prisoners, and they feel aggrieved on this account.

I have noticed that for many people on the island, the prison is largely ignored or forgotten. It is certainly not considered a part of the community which warrants the same amount of attention and support as the hospice. There feels like a degree of embarrassment that we have the the prison here; it provides much-needed work for local people, but that can be seen as the only benefit. As chaplain trying to recruit suitable people to volunteer as prison visitors, it was always a challenge. The same cannot be said of the hospice.

Why is it that prisons and prison staff, who deal with the taboo of crime, are regarded less favourably than a hospice which deals with the taboo of death? It may be partly because death is something that we will all face, and when we are dying or accompanying someone who is, we want there to be good, caring, knowledgeable people around to look after us. So we are committed to ensuring that the hospice is still there when we need it. We are not all going to commit crimes, or to know someone who has, so we are less concerned about prisons, and feel less attachment or responsibility towards them. We know that money to keep them functioning comes from our taxes, but beyond that we have little or no interest in them. It also seems that there is some separation between the deserving and undeserving. If you are dying, you have no choice, and this generates a sympathy and warmth of feeling from others. It draws compassion from people. If you are a prisoner, you have committed an offence, you have broken the rules, and you got what you deserved. People frequently feel condemnation and hostility towards prisoners, especially sex offenders.

The contrast between prisons and hospices in the public eye, is palpable. It is as if the hospice is embraced and adored, idealized and affirmed; while the prison is an embarrassment to the local community. Perhaps prisons are the organizational scapegoat, which pushes to the outside of the community psyche those aspects of ourselves that we would rather deny? Yet the reality is more complex than may first appear. There is a brighter side to the prison, and a darker side to the hospice; recognizing this, naming it and understanding it is a healthier and more wholesome approach for the organizations, for those who work within them and for society as a whole.

Facing the shadow

Both kinds of institutions, prisons and hospices, though very different in function and feeling, provide society with a degree of emotional containment. Prisons contain the dark side of human capabilities, and a hospice contains the dark side of life, death. Both establishments are expert in dealing with and thinking about the taboos which most of the rest of the community avoid. Does their existence help the general population to think about these taboos in a more informed way, or do they take away the responsibility from individuals to do that thinking for themselves? Are prisons and hospices catalysts for education and intelligent thought about these taboos beyond the walls of their buildings?

The containment that a prison provides is both physical and emotional. It contains individuals who have caused others or society harm, but it also represents a container for the shadow or darker side of humanity. Our shadow, which is often in our unconscious mind, is generally what we can't see in ourselves but we recognize more easily in others. The shadow archetype, which Carl Jung conceptualized most fully in the twentieth century, is used as a psychological metaphor to describe the impulses and desires of individuals, their Dr Jekyll and Mr Hyde. It can be applied to organizations as well as to individuals. Perhaps that is why as a society we are less likely to look towards a prison and examine what goes on there. It is so much easier to look away than to look towards what makes us uncomfortable.

Prisons can make prisoners worse: they can learn bad habits from others, or acquire addictions whilst being resident there. Prisons can appear more like "warehouses for the incorrigible than greenhouses for the reformed" (Sir Richard Branson). However, a healthy prison offers prisoners education and training; it provides courses to help prisoners to change attitudes and behaviours. Prison staff can provide excellent role models; they are skilled in defusing situations and professional in the way they deal with prisoners who might be very abusive towards them. There is a strong sense of shared community among the staff and camaraderie and care provided by staff towards one another. There is banter, and a humour which is able to express the darker side of prison life in a lighter manner. (Some of it sails close to the wind!)

A hospice can suffer from chronic niceness and perfectionism and expectations that are unrealistic. At a conference for hospice chaplains, a speaker commented:

> There is a collective fantasy that the staff in a hospice are nice people, who are caring for nice dying people, who are going to have a nice death, in a nice place.

How do hospice staff deal with their actions that are less than perfect or when the people they are caring for are not nice? What if staff cannot make the grade? What if they burn out? Do staff carry the sense of responsibility to be ambassadors for the hospice every hour of the day? Do managers take seriously the emotional strain of dealing with death daily on their staff? How well are staff supported? Where do staff take the projected anger of families who are grieving, or deaths that are messy? What are their behaviours like towards their family and friends? Is there competitiveness within the hospice world to be bigger, better, have a higher rating, make more money, expand its role or save the world from the fear of dying?

An emotionally healthy individual is aware of their darker side, and seeks to integrate and bring to their conscious awareness their impulses and feelings and fears, however unpleasant and challenging they may be. Someone who is able to do this recognizes that they are as capable of harm, even horrendous harm, as anyone else, and yet by recognizing this they are able to make the right moral choices not to act in this way. A term used to describe this kind of approach is "radical honesty". Some prisoners who admit that they have committed great harm have had to recognize the enormity of what they are capable of; they could even be in a more honest self-aware position than some of those who regard them with contempt.

An emotionally healthy organization, whether it is a prison, hospice or another kind of institution, is aware of the darker side of itself. It recognizes the possibility that it may be placing undue pressures on its staff; it sees the potential for being too controlling and micro-managing or too laissez-faire and leaving staff exposed. It sees the potential for cultures of bullying or perfectionism to develop. To mitigate against these dangers, a healthy organization is able to review its function, purpose and ethos and is constantly checking and challenging itself to see that it is living up to its core values; it has good processes and procedures to allow containment of difficult situations and emotions. It encourages reflective practice and does not rush from one project to the next without proper evaluation and due consideration.

A healthy organization welcomes impartial external observation, like that of the Independent Monitoring Board in prisons or trustees in a hospice. It has a culture of inclusion and honesty and allows spaces for the voice of staff at all levels of the organization and service users to be heard.

It recognizes that mistakes may be made, and that learning can happen when they are. It celebrates the contribution and affirms the expertise of its staff; it places a high value on staff support and wellbeing and recognizes the need for people, particularly in demanding face-to-face work, to have external supervision. It encourages staff to be well-rounded individuals and to be boundaried about their work, so that they can have a life and interests beyond it. It recognizes the potential for getting burned out, seeks to minimize this by encouraging staff to take their time off and does not expect them to work over and above their hours. It is able to say thank you and sorry when necessary to individuals or the public.

Facing the shadow in ourselves or in institutions brings into the light the things that are most feared. When the things that are most feared are considered and confronted, they become less frightening. We become more mature, emotionally and spiritually, when we are able to do this. The taboos of criminal behaviours and death often generate fear and avoidance. If we bring these subjects into focus, they become less frightening both to individuals and collectively to society. By facing those taboos, by embracing the shadow of what they represent, they cease to become taboos, and they can be talked about and discussed thoughtfully. Prisons and hospices have an important function to help society break taboos and to bring into the light that which we would otherwise suppress and keep in the dark.

Facing taboos in pastoral care

Simon, who had had cancer for a few years, had come to the hospice following an episode of extreme pain in his shoulders. He had been totally incapacitated and had called out for help, which had not been forthcoming, for half an hour. He lived alone. He thought he was going to die. Eventually he had managed to crawl to a phone and call an ambulance. He was taken to hospital and then transferred to the hospice for further pain management. When Simon told me what had happened to him, he was experiencing symptoms of post-traumatic stress, and every pain he experienced, however minor, made him think it was going to be like the previous incident. He was extremely anxious and frightened. Simon also talked about his diagnosis of cancer, and how he had dealt with it over the last three years. He said that he had taken every opportunity for treatment and chemotherapy; he had really battled against the illness and had told his friends and family that he was coping. They had seemed to applaud him for being strong. Underneath, however, Simon was scared. He admitted that the way he had been presenting himself to his friends and family had been a mask.

When Simon finished talking, I asked if I could share my observations of his experience with him. I put it to him that he had been carrying around this mask for a very long time and that it must have weighed heavily upon him, particularly on his shoulders. I suggested that he had been presenting himself in one way to others (his persona, according to Jung) but that his subconscious mind was trying to awaken him to his real self. His body had to do something dramatic to make him take notice of what was really going on for him; so he was quite literally brought to his knees by the pain. I proposed that if this was the case, then he wouldn't go back to that experience of acute pain again, because he was being real, letting his more vulnerable side emerge and asking for help.

Simon grasped this idea enthusiastically. When I returned to see him the following day, he felt it had been a "light-bulb moment" of revelation. He had slept for the first time in weeks, and he had been able to have conversations with his relatives about making a will and about sensitive family issues that he had never been able to discuss before. Like many people, in my experience especially men, Simon had grown up believing that to express emotion and to ask for help was a sign of weakness. He had felt compelled to use the language of battle against cancer and had put on the armour of the Vikings to do so. One of his hobbies was Viking enactment.

In our second conversation, Simon admitted that because he had been so absorbed addressing his illness, he had never really faced up to the fact that eventually he was going to die. So we began to explore his thoughts and feelings about death. He was not frightened of death itself, but only of how it would happen, and of talking about his wishes to his family. He was worried that it would upset them. Simon could talk to me about death knowing that I was comfortable with discussing it, and he did not have to worry about my feelings. Our conversation about dying gave him confidence to start the conversation with his relatives, and the next day he was able to have a full and frank conversation with his children, using the Advance Care Plan as a guide and focus for this discussion. The Advance Care Plan is a document which enables someone to write down their wishes for care and treatment at the end of life, so that their preferences can be taken into account should they lose the capacity to speak for themselves.

In the space of four days Simon had been transformed. He had embraced the reality of death, and burst the bubble of the taboo. He looked and spoke differently. He had been able to laugh and cry with his family, and now not only had the weight of the mask disappeared, but the weight of the fear of death had also gone. He described himself as liberated. He now looked forward to going home, whereas before he had been scared of doing so; he had had meaningful conversations with the people he cared most about, and he was engaging with other people with greater empathy and wisdom. He was enjoying being this new kind of person, who had thrown away the cape and costume of Superman, as he described it! The benefits of facing the taboos and addressing his shadow had not only been for himself, but his family shared it too. They described feeling easier now that they had been able to talk about their father's death rather than avoiding discussing it completely.

This pastoral encounter confirmed for me once again the necessity and value of breaking the taboo of death. In our last conversation at the hospice, Simon said he was keen to go home and get on with living for however long or short that might be. I told him that another patient had said to me that she was living most fully now that she was dying. This statement resonated strongly with Simon's experience. I asked him if I might include his story in this book. He was delighted to think that by sharing how he had broken the taboo of death he might be able to help someone else.

Theological reflection

The death of Jesus is such a central element of the Christian story that one might imagine that talking about death and dying would come easily to people who follow this faith. Colleagues in parish ministry have told me that death is still a taboo amongst their congregations, and that if they preach about dying, some people will complain! My observations from working with people who are dying and their families show a complex picture. There are many whose faith gives them a hope in the resurrection and a belief in life after death, but that does not necessarily mean that they will be comfortable in talking about their own or their loved one's mortality. Faith may bring comfort in the face of death, but it may have little impact on the taboo of death itself.

If we look at the Gospels, particularly John 13–16, much of Jesus' teaching of his closest friends is to prepare them for his impending death. Here, Jesus is talking to his disciples:

> Then he began to teach them that the Son of Man must undergo great suffering, and be rejected by the elders, the chief priests, and the scribes, and be killed, and after three days rise again. He said all this quite openly.
>
> *Mark 8.31–33*

This uncomfortable conversation is challenged by Peter. We don't know the content of what Peter says, but we can imagine that he is probably telling Jesus not to be so negative, that his talk is morbid and depressing and that it will get the group down, and that Jesus should be more optimistic. What we do hear is Jesus' vehement response to Peter, in front of all the disciples: "Get behind me, Satan! You are a stumbling block to me; for you are setting your mind not on divine things but on human things" (Mark 8:33b).

Jesus is clear. Facing suffering and death is of God; failing to do so is not. Shortly after this episode in Mark's Gospel, Jesus again talks about his death (Mark 9.30), but his disciples do not understand, and we are told that they are afraid to ask. Perhaps the vehemence of Jesus' earlier reaction to Peter makes them even more afraid. Even in the time of Jesus people still found it hard to talk about death, and the disciples who were closest to Jesus, and who loved him the most, found it hardest of all.

Jesus constantly confronted the taboos of society. He reached out to those who were considered to taint others by their presence; lepers, those who were mentally disturbed, women. He recognized the suffering these individuals experienced, and saw beyond the labels and restrictions that others had placed upon them. Jesus frequently challenged the religious and law-abiding who considered themselves righteous and who held themselves aloof from the people that Jesus was drawn to. He said: "Those who are well have no need of a physician, but those who are sick; I have come to call not the righteous but sinners to repentance" (Luke 5:31–32).

When Jesus went to the synagogue in his home town of Nazareth, he chose to read from the prophet Isaiah:

> The Spirit of the Lord is upon me,
> because he has anointed me
> to bring good news to the poor.
> He has sent me to proclaim release to the captives
> and recovery of sight to the blind,
> to let the oppressed go free,
> to proclaim the year of the Lord's favour.
>
> *Luke 4:18–19*

Jesus clearly identifies himself with this calling, and his ministry with those whom society ostracizes and considers taboo; the poor, the outcast, the prisoner, the oppressed. These were the people who knew their need for God, who recognized their own brokenness and who were more aware of their darker side than those who thought of themselves as holy.

> And he rolled up the scroll, gave it back to the attendant, and sat down. The eyes of all in the synagogue were fixed on him.Then he began to say to them, "Today this scripture has been fulfilled in your hearing".
>
> *Luke 4:20–21*

In the Beatitudes (Matthew 5:3–12), Jesus challenges what society considers to be blessings—wealth, prosperity, avoidance of pain and suffering. Instead, he tells his hearers that the ones who are blessed are those who mourn and those who are persecuted. In my experience of journeying with those who go through times of great trial and who have to face head-on the reality of bereavement, or loss, or the fear of death, are the people who develop depths and insights which those whose lives are without struggle may never encounter. There are surprising and extraordinary blessings in experiencing life and death in this way. Jesus also says, "Blessed are the meek." In our language, we associate meekness with weakness, and putting up with things, or in colloquial language of being like a "doormat". This is not the intention from the Greek, the language in which this passage was first written. Someone who is meek recognizes their power, they hold a sword in their possession, and they know that they could use it for harm. A meek person chooses not to use this weapon or their power in this way, they keep the sword sheathed. In the same way a person who has considered the shadow side and acknowledges their power, but who chooses not to exercise it, is blessed, and will inherit the earth.

In the final week of Jesus' life, Jesus himself becomes taboo. He is arrested as a criminal, beaten as an offender and killed for being a blasphemer. He is on the outside of the religious and societal rules of his day. In doing so, does he not take away the sting, not only of death itself but of the other taboos with which he is associated? Jesus' arrest, trial, death and resurrection challenge the power of the taboo through the real human experience of God.

CHAPTER 10

Lessons Learned

In the previous chapter I reflected on the importance for individuals and society of breaking the taboos associated with imprisonment and death. I shall look further at this in the final chapter as I consider what I have learned from the people I have accompanied into the depths of pain and suffering.

Facing being in prison, or facing death, be it our own or that of someone close to us, remind us that we are not in control. We are confronted by the reality that we are in a situation that we can do little to change. For many people this may be the first time that this has happened to them. For the rest of their lives they have decided where to live, who to have as friends, what job to do, when to go to bed, how to use their leisure. Being very ill or coming to prison strips many of those choices away. How someone faces and deals with this lack of control varies according to their personality and previous life experiences. Someone whose life has been chaotic due to drug or alcohol addiction may welcome the structure of prison life; someone who has held a responsible job or who has given commands to others may find it very hard to accept that their physical condition means they now need help to do the basic tasks.

When I first started working at HMP Holloway, I was struck by the importance of not taking anything for granted. Prisoners were handed plates and cups and cutlery to use when they first arrived in custody. The cups were blue plastic and had the stains of previous owners' hot drinks in them that no amount of washing could eradicate. It made the drinks all taste similar, an odd mixture of tea, coffee, hot chocolate and soup. When I went home and drank my own tea from a china mug, I noticed it and valued it in a completely different way. This small detail of life in prison gave me an insight into prison life that few have the opportunity to consider. It reminded me that the cost of imprisonment on the grand scale is about the loss of freedom and control, but on the small scale it is also the loss of a decent cup of tea.

Working in a hospice has also taught me appreciation. Life can end very suddenly and when we least expect it, so to value the time that we have by enjoying and living it to the full is the best way to live. This is not the same as the idea of "eat, drink and be merry for tomorrow we die". It is much more profound and positive than this. It is recognizing by using all of our senses the beauty that surrounds us; it is appreciating what we have rather than craving more and more; it is valuing and investing in our relationships with others and living compassionately; it is being able to flourish and thrive as who we really are and not how we think others want us to be.

Many people don't see this, sadly, and live their unhappy lives waiting for the time when they can enjoy things, not really knowing or appreciating what they do have until it is too late. I remember being shocked when talking to a prison officer in his early twenties who knew to the day when he would be retiring from his job in forty years, and who was looking forward to this time when he could start to enjoy himself! In the meantime his life was slipping by, and he barely noticed it. As John Lennon sang in his song "Beautiful boy", "Life is what happens to you while you're busy making other plans."

Living in the present

The maxim *carpe diem*, "seize the day", doesn't go far enough when you work in a hospice, or are with people who are dying. You have to seize the moment, because there may not be another. This is a wonderful way to live life, as it encourages us to take opportunities when they are presented, and to make the most of the now. This is a valuable lesson for living that death can teach us. I have spent years telling myself that I will write my reflections on ministry down, and it is now, as I confront the reality of my own mortality more fully through my work in the hospice, that I am doing what I have put off for so long. If we have things that we want to do, or things that we need to say to others, we should not put it off, for one of the hardest things to come to terms with when one is dying, or when facing the death of someone who has died unexpectedly, is having to live with regrets.

When I was a chaplain in a busy local prison, Holloway, where the average length of stay for prisoners was 28 days, I learned very quickly that I had to make each conversation significant. As chaplains we were required by statute to see all the new arrivals to the prison within twenty-four hours. The woman we saw one day as a remand prisoner could be returned to court the next, and we would never see her again; or a prisoner could be sent to another prison very quickly once sentenced. So every conversation counted, even if it were for a very short period of time. In the same way, working in the hospice has taught me that you have to respond very quickly to requests from a patient or family member.

One morning as I headed to a meeting in our hospice day-centre I was accosted by a doctor and nurse from the ward. The previous evening a patient had expressed her desire to get married to her partner of many years. They had always joked that they would tie the knot when they were on their deathbeds. It was clear that Julie did not have long to live. In some slight panic I realized that it would come to me to sort out the necessary arrangements. Fortunately, a colleague at the hospital who had previously been the chaplain at the hospice was at the end of the phone to give me advice and guidance. Every other planned activity for that morning was put aside, as I made the necessary phone calls to the registrar and drew up paperwork. While I was doing that, others had gone shopping for flowers, balloons and banners, someone had been to the hospice shop to get suitable shirts for bride and groom, and the consultant had arranged for the correct dosage of drugs to enable the bride to be alert for as long as possible. By 3.30 p.m. the registrar was in place, and the civil ceremony took place with the consultant as one of the witnesses. The couple then decided that they would like a religious blessing, so cancelling a day's leave for the following day I took the service. This time about fifteen local friends from the bowling club came to witness and support them both. It was incredibly moving. Julie died three days later.

When I worked in a women's prison, a probation officer, a counsellor and I devised a course to support and assist women who were in prison for the first time. It was a small group lasting for six sessions and covered coping skills and relaxation techniques, as well as giving the women the space and security to talk about their feelings of coming to prison and the problems they faced there. In one session, we looked at our methods of thinking, highlighting diagrammatically that for many of us our thoughts swing like a pendulum: from the past—memories good and bad, regrets, experiences—to the future—what will I do, how will it be when I get old? Both regrets about the past and worries about the future can generate strong feelings. Swinging backwards and forwards in our thoughts can be extremely exhausting, emotionally draining and, ultimately, debilitating. What we encouraged participants on the course to recognize was that the past has already happened and we cannot return there, and the future has not happened yet, so there is no point in worrying about something that may never come to pass.

The only place you can fully inhabit is the present moment. Noticing our own thought processes and nudging ourselves back to focus on the present moment and living fully in it, not only gives us a greater awareness and appreciation of what we have right in front of us, but it also gives us back control, not of our outward circumstances, but of how we choose to think about them.

Prayer and silence

Meditation and contemplative prayer use the breath as a focus for staying in the here and now. Our breath is with us until we take our last breath with death; we can use breath to connect us to the movement of the body, and slowing our breathing can bring us to a place of calm and inner silence. The way of contemplation is found in many faiths and spiritual practices, and it is part of the Christian tradition. Through working in a hospice and developing my own spiritual practices, I am more convinced that learning to be comfortable in silence is the best way of preparing ourselves for death itself. As one moves into the final stages of life, there is less and less need or opportunity for conversation, and more and more space for silence. The more one practises quieting the mind from endless chatter, the more one is drawn into the hidden depths of tranquillity. Rabbi Rami Shapiro, teacher, writer and broadcaster on religion and spirituality says, "the deepest language of the soul is silence".

Martin Laird, in his book *Into the Silent Land*, talks of the silence of contemplation as being as the place of encounter with God who is the ground of our being. He describes silence as the "urgent necessity",[10] if we are to hear God speaking in the eternal silence in which we are all connected. Laird talks of the spiritual practice of silence not as a technique but as a way of life and being which draws us deeply into awareness of ourselves; enables us to become witnesses to our thoughts and distractions rather than victims of them; and which allows us to move beyond judgement of ourselves or others. It permits us to experience our own vulnerability and see beyond the limits of our pain and suffering.

Suffering as mystery and growth

How we think about pain and suffering will affect how we approach death, our own or another's. The Buddhist tradition sees suffering as part of the inevitability of living. I find this helpful. If we search for a kind of existence which avoids all pain, we are going to be disappointed; if we embrace suffering as an opportunity to develop inner strengths or to learn wisdom, then our perspective changes and we are more able to find acceptance and peace.

Sheila Cassidy and Elisabeth Kübler-Ross both worked in palliative care for many years and have written extensively about their experiences. Cassidy distinguishes between suffering as problem and suffering as mystery. Suffering as problem suggests that there is a solution, a call to action which motivates us; for example, the challenge to work for justice for those who are poor and marginalized, campaigning for the homeless and destitute, providing hospitals and medication for the sick. This is active compassion. Suffering as mystery encompasses the cries from the heart, why me? There is no action to this kind of suffering; there is only standing alongside another with compassion and empathy, whilst holding on to hope and belief.

Kübler-Ross wrote a book called *Death, the Final Stage of Growth*. The very title challenges the notion that everything about death is negative. I have shared the title of this book with people who are at the end of their lives, and it has struck a chord with many. I have witnessed people make massive transformations as they have drawn closer to death; by becoming more compassionate; by letting go of past hurts; by making peace with others or with themselves. I have seen frightened people become brave, and victims become survivors. I have seen people whose lives have been pretty ordinary become extraordinary. I have seen bullies become vulnerable, cynics find faith in humanity, even atheists find faith in God. There is no doubt in my mind that dying is an extraordinary business. If the persona can be left behind, then there is room for the whole person to be revealed in all their glory. Perhaps as the one who is dying faces the taboo of death and finds it something to be embraced rather than feared then, like Simon in Chapter 9, they can feel liberated finally to be themselves.

One woman who had been terrified of dying and of leaving this life behind said shortly before she died, "I suppose I could look at dying as an adventure!" When someone makes this breakthrough for themselves, I can only describe it as a moment of joy and celebration, a moment of holiness. It leaves me wanting to pump my fist in the air with delight and cry out, "Yes! You have made it! Alleluia!"

I have never ceased to be astonished at the strength of the human spirit. I have learned again and again from those I have met that people can and do survive the most complex of experiences. The courage and hope in humanity that has been instilled in me has empowered me to be able to hold on to the possibility of transformation in the next person I meet in distress or pain. However, I never make comparisons from one situation to another, or tell someone that somebody else has worked through this kind of pain so they should too; rather it is a quiet confidence within me that people are often stronger than they imagine they are, and given the right set of circumstances, patience and insight, others too may find meaning and hope in their experiences.

Esther was one of the most courageous women that I met in prison. She had been an outspoken critic of a political leader in her home country in Africa and had been sent to prison as a political prisoner. This was after her father had been burned alive in front of her, and her children and mother had disappeared. She had no idea whether or not they were still alive. She had escaped from prison by bribing the guards and had walked across her country's border to a neighbouring country. Here she received a false passport and fled to Britain. She survived for a short time living on the streets, before being arrested for trying to leave the country with false documentation. She faced being deported back to her country of origin.

It is hard to imagine the torment of grief and sorrow in Esther's life, but you would never guess her story by her demeanour. She was always dignified, compassionate, generous and cheerful, and any moments of despair or grief she permitted herself were short-lived and fought with determination. She had a strong Christian faith which sustained her despite her distressing circumstances. While I am a great advocate for keeping emotional boundaries, I am not always able to maintain the standards I set. Esther's story affected me deeply, and I and others tried to support her in her legal case to remain in the UK and to get bail. We were not successful. She was removed from prison to await deportation in a detention centre. I went to visit her there. While I felt enraged at the injustice of Esther's situation, and dismayed that she would have to return to her country probably to be imprisoned again, or even killed, Esther's resilience, courage and faith was inspiring and deeply humbling. I have no idea what happened to her when she returned home.

We can never really know what our response will be to an experience of suffering until we have to face it. Neither can we presume to anticipate how someone else might experience their pain. Anita is locked into her body due to Motor Neurone Disease. She is totally dependent on others to assist her, with moving, eating, washing, toileting. She communicates now by a piece of equipment with which, by slight movement, she can type out letters onto a screen using a censor on her forehead. Previously she held a responsible job and managed her own affairs. To hear of her situation, one might assume that she would be depressed, angry, hostile, self-pitying; most of us would think we would be like this if we were in her position. Anita is not. Perhaps she has had or still does have moments of despair, but it is hard to imagine. She is bright-eyed and radiant. She laughs frequently with an infectious giggle that gets everyone in the hospice day-centre laughing alongside. She used to do laughter therapy every morning for thirty minutes in her garden in Asia, she tells me! Well, it works, and she is teaching all of us who meet her the importance of humour, for it means that her life-limiting and degenerative condition has not got the better of her spirit, for she will have the last laugh!

Neil had been in prison for nearly three decades when I first met him; heavily bearded and a little stooped, he looked like a mixture of an Old Testament prophet and Father Christmas! He was still in a Category B prison, and there didn't seem much prospect of him ever being released. Most of us would think that he would be desperate and despondent, feeling that his life had been a total waste and without meaning. I have no doubt that Neil had experienced these feelings in the earlier part of his time in prison. He had great empathy for the youngsters who were coming in who tried to battle the prison system in a vain effort to make sense of their situation and themselves. But somewhere along the route of years incarcerated Neil had discovered artistic talents and produced some fine paintings, including one of the crucifixion. He was happier than he had ever been before, he was comfortable with the person he had become, and he was full of gratitude for the things that life had given him, as well as having a heartfelt concern for others in worse situations than himself. He had also found faith and solace in the quiet of the Quaker tradition; from a way of violence he had discovered the path to peace.

These people, and countless others whom I have met, have managed somehow to transform their situation of suffering from despair to hope, from catastrophe to enlightenment. I would probably say through grace, certainly through a great deal of hard inner work and soul-searching.

Connectivity and community

When people are faced with loss, pain, suffering, they are often stronger than they would have imagined they could be or they discover skills of survival and coping which they were unaware they had. How they find these gifts is something of a mystery. However, I believe it often comes from feeling connected to others.

People in prison or a hospice are gathered together, not out of choice, but because of adversity. Within that suffering community there will be a vast range of circumstances and attitudes to their condition. This sense of community can have a profound effect. Sometimes it comes from seeing others coping with similar situations that gives inspiration. Sometimes seeing others in a worse situation can help people to put their own in perspective. I have noticed that many find comfort and healing in helping others. In prison I have seen many prisoners, who have really struggled to come to terms with being there, later volunteer to be Listeners; by offering help to prisoners in distress they know that they are doing something of value and meaning. Bereaved relatives often choose to volunteer in the hospice for similar reasons.

I have observed that when one person who is struggling with their own pain or loss begins to recognize and empathize with the suffering of another person, or group, then there is a shift from darkness towards the light. Ken was dying; he had experienced a great deal of physical and emotional pain, but on watching the news he was distressed seeing the suffering of the children in Syria; by feeling compassion and empathy for them he was able to see that at least he had had a good life, and that their situation was more desperate than his. This is a kind of realignment of oneself away from the centre to the sidelines, and making somebody else the focus of one's attention and sympathy. In doing this Ken was becoming part of a world of suffering, a community of people across the world and throughout history who had or were experiencing pain. He felt a sense of connection which he had not previously known.

People who are terminally ill but living at home can come to the hospice daycentre for medical, practical, emotional and social support. When someone from the hospice day services dies, we hold a memorial event for them using poems and music that the person liked and sharing memories of them. As well as honouring the person and recognizing their uniqueness and legacy, it is also a way of connecting us all together, staff, volunteers and patients. We are acknowledging the reality of our own mortality but restating our value to each other as part of a community.

People who have been bereaved can feel very isolated and lonely, feeling that friends and neighbours avoid them or that their sadness makes them socially taboo. They can feel abnormal and wonder if their grief is making them go mad. Bereaved people can find support when they hear that other grieving people have similar experiences and feelings. Sharing these feelings in groups or with other bereaved individuals can be very helpful. Finding kindred spirits who have experienced loss themselves, and yet who are progressing through their journey of grief, can be of great encouragement.

As I approached people to ask their permission to write about them in this book, I found not only a willingness and enthusiasm from people to be included, but a strong sense that by agreeing to this they were going to be enabling someone else to benefit from their experiences. I have noticed so many people finding redemption from self-pity and guilt by feeling that they have something to pass on to others. I frequently draw attention to this in pastoral conversations of any kind; not only reminding each person that they are teaching me something, which I can then pass on to someone else, but demonstrating the connectedness of our human experience, and that all our encounters with one another are part of a web of meaning and hope in which we all dwell.

Theological reflection

When people are confronted with suffering, loss, pain and grief in their life I find them asking questions such as how can a loving God allow the person I love to go through this kind of pain? Why doesn't God do something? Can there even be a God, if God seems not to answer when I call for help? These are the spiritual pains of someone who is in pain or witnessing the pain of one they love.

These questions are not new. They are probably as old as suffering itself, and in every age, every philosophy, every faith they have been wrestled with. The whole of the book of Job, in the Hebrew scriptures, and in the Christian Old Testament, is concerned with the matter of how a good person suffers and whether or not there is any reason or meaning in it.

Why doesn't an all-powerful God do something to change the world? Does God sit by and watch us make a mess of everything? Does God simply send us suffering to see how we get on with it, thinking up more and more extreme forms to find our breaking point? Is this some divine comedy, or a calculated game of chess in which humanity always loses?

If this is the kind of God that any of the faiths preach, no wonder people are put off and call themselves atheists. This is a tyrant and despot, one not worthy of praise and thanksgiving, but of condemnation and anger.

Even as a young child I thought about these difficult questions, and they have stayed with me into adulthood. If I have found any answers they have been from my experiences and in the recounting of the narrative of Holy Week. I feel that I have worked in very "Good Friday" places, and I have sometimes wondered if I can ever move on from the Passion story. Do I remain forever in the sadness and sorrow of the crucifixion? Can I really believe in the hope of the resurrection? Whenever I am tempted to doubt the other part of the Holy Week events, usually something or generally someone reminds me of the hope that lies beyond the sorrow. Perhaps it will be Esther, who faced her deportation back to an uncertain future with calm; or Tina, who found her voice in the face of death and let go of her anger; or Angela, with Parkinson's and cancer, who feels her body diminishing daily and said recently, "As my body becomes more fragile, my spirit becomes stronger."

It is these experiences of "little resurrections" which remind me time and time again that suffering and pain, and death itself, are not the end of the story. It is the people I have worked with who have found in themselves courage, hope, self-worth, peace and healing, that have taught me to continue to have faith in the resurrection.

When I enter imaginatively into the story of the first Easter morning, when Mary Magdalene goes to Jesus' tomb, I witness the depths and turmoil of loss and bereavement which anyone who has lost someone they love experiences. Here is a woman whose life has been transformed by her love of Jesus. She has devoted herself to him and trusted him in a way she has never trusted anyone before. She has discovered in him the true meaning of love, and now she is experiencing the cost. She is beside herself with grief. She has watched, helpless, as her beloved has been tortured and killed with no justification. She will be forever traumatized as she hears the sound of the nails hammered into his hands or listens to his groans of pain from the cross.

She feels enraged with the disciples for not protecting him, with the crowds for being so fickle, with the religious authorities for being so blindly jealous, with Jesus himself for leaving her, with God for not stepping in to save him. She is angry with herself for ever getting involved with Jesus and putting herself through all this pain now. She is exhausted from replaying the last few days over and over in her mind and unpacking the never-ending "if onlys". She alternates between anger and numbness. She didn't know there were so many feelings she could experience, or that she could switch from one to another with such speed and force. She is exhausted, and yet she cannot sleep; sick to the stomach and unable to eat. She is despairing for life continuing but wants this unbearable pain to cease. She had no idea that she could cry so much; would the tears never stop? But does she really want them to end because that would mean she was getting over it, and she doesn't want that either? She has no idea what to do with herself, she has no notion of how she can survive without him.

It was in this turbulent state of emotional chaos and confusion that Mary went to the tomb. Here she felt she might get some comfort by being physically close to Jesus' body. At least she could perhaps talk to him away from everyone else, perhaps it would give her some relief? But the horror of the situation worsens further, when she sees the stone rolled away and the body stolen. How could anyone do this? Could people not even let his poor broken body rest in peace? This was desecration. It was despicable. She had thought it couldn't get any worse but it just did. In further agony, despondency and rage, she hurries back to the others to tell them the news. Then, wearier than ever, blinded by this latest insult to her beloved, she trudges back to the tomb. Her head and eyes ache, she feels decades older than her years, she stumbles and falls at the entrance of the tomb and wails an unearthly cry of grief. She could be angry with men who are sitting there who ask her why she is crying. She could scream at them, don't you know? Don't you care? Why does the world carry on like this? Why does the sun continue to shine and the birds still sing? It is an insult to her grief! But she has no more energy to be angry now, she is exhausted beyond anything she has ever known.

Then there is someone else there, she assumes he is the gardener. A last surge of desperate energy as she thinks he might have taken the body. Perhaps he can tell her where Jesus is? Tell me, please, please, she begs through her blinding tears. "Mary," he says. She recognizes that voice. Her heart seems to stop, her breath held mid-gasp. It can't be. I must be dreaming. This is another cruel trick that sorrow is playing on me. I am going mad. The thoughts tumble over one another in an instant. Then at last she recognizes him, at last she sees and believes: "Teacher!" Then the transformation from sorrow to joy; despair to ecstasy; doubt to faith.

It is this immense change in Mary and the other disciples that keeps me believing in Jesus' resurrection. It has no rational explanation. It is best described as a mystery. However, it is what helps me hold on to hope, when all seems hopeless; it helps me look beyond the immediate situation of darkness to see a glimmer of light ahead. Frequently, I don't share my Christian faith with the people I meet; often there is no need, and it may not be appropriate. What I think I convey is the assurance that I have hope in them, and for them; that meaning may emerge from their experience and that whatever happens they are held in the loving embrace of one who understands their pain.

We cannot avoid pain and suffering; it is an inevitable part of the human condition. Nor can we get away from death and dying, and if we have risked loving others during our lives, leave-taking hurts. But the resurrection story, and the experiences of people I have accompanied into the depths of darkness who have emerged into the light, give me the assurance that suffering and death do not have the last word, that love triumphs in the end. Sheila Cassidy writes:

> I believe that our spiritual attitude to suffering is crucial because it not only determines the way we relate to those for whom we care but our very survival as carers. . . . If . . . we are able to maintain a paschal overview, keeping the resurrection in the same perspective as the cross, then our inevitable human sadness will be tempered by the joy we experience in our faith in the loving purpose of God.[11]

Some of this book has been written while I have been staying in a convent in Southsea in Portsmouth, with a small community of Anglican nuns, the Sisters of Bethany. The chapel window, designed and engraved by artist Tracey Sheppard, is plain glass except for the cross which fills the central panel. If you come into the chapel in the night-time when the chapel lights are on, the window is dark and the cross stands out. On the cross the words "I am the resurrection and the life" are engraved—"resurrection" fills the horizontal beam. When you see the window in the daytime, you realize that the etching is not of the cross itself, but only of its outline. The cross itself is clear glass, and through it you can see the beauty of the garden beyond. Seen in this light, the cross is always present, but it has become a part, not the whole, of the bigger scene of beauty.

I see this window as a wonderful theological symbol. In the darkness of our suffering we can only see the cross and the pain; we hold on to the hope of the resurrection, but we fail to grasp its meaning. When the light dawns, we can see through the cross and glimpse Life beyond. The panel of glass separating the chapel from the garden, inside from out, is like the thin separation between death and life, through which we must all pass. It is the cross, the symbol of pain, torture and death, which dominates our consciousness when we are in the darkness, experiencing our own pain or witnessing the pain of others. But when the daylight comes, our perspective changes, and though we can still see the cross, it is now part, not the whole, of the window. Beyond the pain, through the cross, we can see beauty and life that awaits us.

> Death is not the extinguishing of the light, it is putting out the lamp because the dawn has come.
>
> *Rabindranath Tagore*

Bibliography

Albom, Mitch, *The Timekeeper* (London: Sphere, 2012).

Buber, Martin, *I and Thou* (New York: Simon and Schuster; 1st Touchstone edition, 2008).

Cassidy, Sheila, *Sharing the Darkness* (London: Darton, Longman and Todd, 1988).

Dostoevsky, Fyodor, *The House of the Dead* (London: J. M. Dent & Sons Ltd, 1911).

Du Boulay, Shirley with Rankin, Marianne, *Cicely Saunders The Founder of the Modern Hospice Movement* (London: SPCK, 2007).

Hughes, Gerald, *Walk to Jerusalem* (London: Darton, Longman and Todd, 1991).

Kübler-Ross, Elisabeth, *Death, The Final Stage of Growth* (New York: Simon and Schuster, Inc., 1975).

Kübler-Ross, Elisabeth, *On Death and Dying* 40th Anniversary Edition (London: Routledge, 2009).

Laird, Martin, *Into the Silent Land: The Practice of Contemplation* (London: Darton, Longman and Todd, 2006).

Lewis, C. S., *A Grief Observed* (London: Faber and Faber, 1966).

Murray Parkes, Colin, *Bereavement, Studies in Grief in Adult Life* New Edition (London: Penguin Books, 1996).

Nouwen, Henri, *The Wounded Healer* (New York: Crown Publishing Group, 1979).

Pattison, Stephen, *A Critique of Pastoral Care* (London: SCM Press Ltd, 1988).

Rohr, Richard, *The Divine Dance* (London: SPCK, 2016).

Royal College of Physicians, *Talking about Dying* (19 October 2018).

Storr, Anthony, *Jung* (London: Fontana Paperbacks, 1973).

Tagore, Rabindranath, *Gitanjali: Song Offerings* (New York: Simon and Schuster, 1997).

Vanstone, W. H., *The Stature of Waiting* (London: Darton, Longman and Todd, 1982).

Ward, Tess, *Alternative Pastoral Prayers* (Norwich: Canterbury Press, 2012).

Winnicott, Donald, *Playing and Reality* (London: Routledge; 2nd Edition, 2005).

Notes

[1] Stephen Pattison, *A Critique of Pastoral Care* (London: SCM Press, 1988), p. 16.

[2] Martin Buber, *I and Thou* (New York: Simon and Schuster, 2008), p. 11.

[3] Gerard W. Hughes, *Walk to Jerusalem* (London: Darton, Longman and Todd Ltd, 1991), p. 28.

[4] Harvey Gillman, *Criminal Justice*, panel of Quaker Tapestry exhibited in Kendal, Cumbria, UK.

[5] Colin Murray Parkes, *Bereavement, Studies of Grief in Adult Life*, New Edition (London: Penguin, 1998), p. 26.

[6] C. S. Lewis, *A Grief Observed* (London: Faber and Faber Ltd, 1961), p. 5.

[7] Murray Parkes, *Bereavement*, p. 6.

[8] Richard Rohr, *The Divine Dance* (London: SPCK, 2016), p. 103.

[9] Report from the Royal College of Physicians, October 2018.

[10] Martin Laird, *Into the Silent Land* (London: Darton, Longman and Todd, 2006), p. 2.

[11] Sheila Cassidy, *Sharing the Darkness* (London: Darton, Longman and Todd, 1988), p. 64.